WILD
BEAUTY

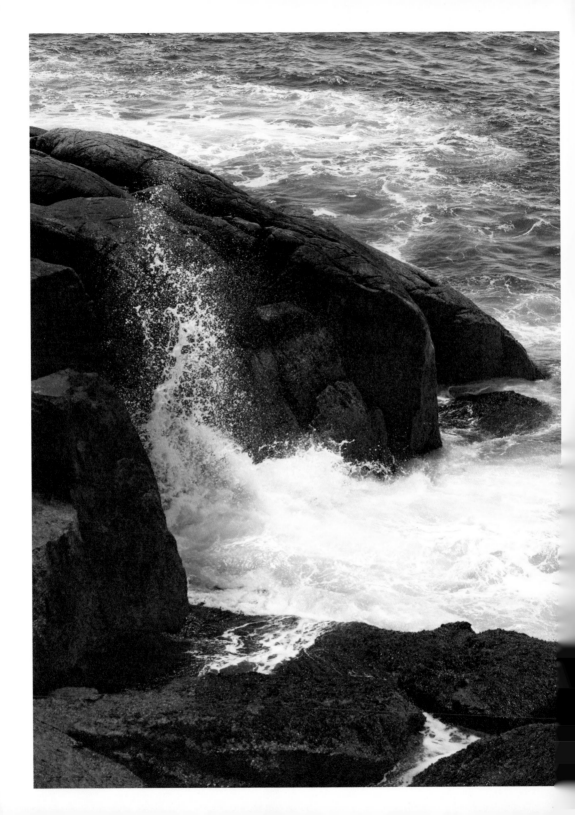

WILD
BEAUTY

wisdom & recipes
for natural self-care

JANA BLANKENSHIP
Foreword by Mandy Aftel

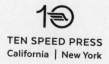

TEN SPEED PRESS
California | New York

Contents

Foreword 7

INTRODUCTION
Captain's Log 8

CHAPTER ONE
Trusting Your Nose 16

The Heart of Plants 19

Hydrosols 22

Scent Extractions 22

Carriers 28

Aromatherapy 29

Primal Magic 32

CHAPTER TWO
Aromatics 34

Base Notes 37

Middle Notes 38

Top Notes 43

Essential Oils During Pregnancy 45

Vine Jamine Blend 49

Vernal Neroli Blend 50

Venus Rose Blend 50

Loosen the Knot
Tension-Release Blend 53

Sweet Rest Calming Blend 54

Forest Sprite Grounding Blend 54

Deep Breath Calming Spray 57

Emerald Green Woods Room Spray 57

Good Vibrations Clearing Spray 58

CHAPTER THREE
Pursuing Wild Beauty 60

Demystifying Ingredient Lists 63

Ingredients I Love 67

Ingredients to Avoid 72

Emerald Sea Detox Bath 77

Aquamarine Bubble Bath 77

Hydrating Body Wash 78

No-More-Scales Body Oil 79

Dream-Cream Deodorant 80

Cocoa-Nut Body Butter 82

Fly & Tick Spray 83

Sea Salt & Sunshine Body Scrub 84

CHAPTER FOUR

Skin 86

Oil Essentials 88
Treating Dry Skin 89

Collagen & Elastin 91

Cocoa & Spice Face Mask & Exfoliant 96
Fresh Face Fruit Mask: 4 Variations 99
Maine Face Mask 100
Clean Slate Makeup Remover
& Oil-Based Cleanser 100
Creamy Shea Face Cleanser 103
Fresh Green Tea Clarifying Toner 105

Smell the Roses Face Toner
& Body Mist 106
Golden Glow Face Balm 108
Deep Sleep Eye Serum 109
Butterfly Daytime Face Oil 110
Lick Your Lips Balm 113
Shimmer & Pop Highlighter 114

CHAPTER FIVE

Hair 116

Taking Care of Hair 118

Mermaid Hair Mask 120
Milk & Honey Shampoo 122
Refreshing Hibiscus ACV Rinse 123
Shining Waves Hair Oil 125

Sea Salt Wave Spray 126
Witchy Coconut Leave-In
Conditioner & Detangler 126
Sail-Away Dry Shampoo 127

CHAPTER SIX

Wild Nature 128

Self Care 132
Gratitude 134

Herbal Allies & Medicinal Foods 137

Green Beauty Juice 140
Mer-Made Energy Drink 143
Golden Glow Elixir 144
Summer Sun Garden Tea 147
Green Sprite Tea 147

Wild Beauty Tea 148
Petal Tea 149
Rose & Coconut Water 150
Superpower Cocoa Mix 150

Afterword 153
Acknowledgments 154
Resources 156

Bibliography 157
Notes 157
Index 158

In memory of Peter G. Cook and Thea Duell.

To my mom Ljiljana, my dad Peter,
and my brother Sasa, for your love and support.
To my husband Levi, my anchor,
and my children Mila and Caspian, my joy.

Foreword

I love *Wild Beauty*! It is beautiful, inspiring, accessible, and full of an infectious spirit of discovery. Jana Blankenship is the perfect guide to show you the best possible way to make something with natural aromatics and plant-based ingredients, for yourself or as a gift. She writes with such ease and grace, and provides simple but foolproof instructions. There is a wealth of information for making body products, room sprays, facial treatments, and scrubs presented in this delightful book.

If you've ever thought you might like to just mix even a few essential oils together and make something, this is the book for you. Reading this book is like having a treasured friend take you by the hand and introduce you to something wonderful. Making things with natural essences is both fun and deeply satisfying. I promise that you will find working with essential oils lifts your mood and makes your heart happy. Natural aromas and materials connect us to our essential selves and to the wild and beautiful natural world. Let Jana bring more of that into your life: with *Wild Beauty*, you will learn to follow your nose as it leads you into a world of delight and happiness.

MANDY AFTEL
Natural perfumer, teacher, and author

Captain's Log

"Beauty is pervasive, inspiration is pervasive." [1]

Agnes Martin, *Writings*

I was a kid who loved to make potions; maybe you were, too? Pine needles, grass, rose petals, mint, anything that smelled and looked good growing in our yard was fodder for my creations. I concocted odd-colored tinctures and tried unsuccessfully to feed them to my family.

I grew up in Cambridge, Massachusetts, and my mother, Ljiljana, was a fashion designer. She would go to couture shows and return home with bottles of perfume to add to her collection. It was the mid-1980s; perfume was decadent, exhilarating, and entirely synthetic. I was mesmerized by her mirrored vanity filled with bottles of all colors, shapes, and smells. They all possessed alluring names, like Opium, Obsession, and Poison. She didn't care about these intriguing bottles, so she let me play tiny chemist. I would mix the perfumes together into my own "signature" scents. I still have the first one I made, which I called "Scents of Hawaii." The name is written in an eight-year-old's handwriting on a white office label pasted on an old Giorgio bottle. Almost thirty years later, it still smells as strongly of Giorgio. If you buried it and dug it up in five thousand years, I think its scent would still be as pervasive.

This innocent, heavy mixing as a child changed my life. I developed a sensitivity to synthetic fragrances and abandoned my love of scent. I steered clear of the beauty departments at shopping malls, and if I did get a whiff of your Teen Spirit, it gave me a visceral reaction that resulted in a headache and nausea. I used everything fragrance-free until my midtwenties, when I smelled an exquisite natural perfume that awakened my lost olfactory passion. From then on, I discovered natural perfumery and the rich palette of essential oils. I studied soapmaking, explored herbalism, and ended up changing career paths from curating art to curating scents. The childhood love of making potions turned into making natural beauty products in my home for fun and then starting my own budding business.

As I look back on my path, I see signs along the way that led me to this place. I had a background in the arts; I was a painter and then became a curator. However, I never thought in my wildest dreams I would start a business. But as I turn back the pages, I see my mother during my youth, her office full of soft piles of her creations, wool sweaters, and hand-dyed silk dresses. My mother traveled around the world to bring these works to life: yarn from Iceland, silk from China, production in Serbia. As a child, I witnessed the web she wove, a creative life that cloaked people in warmth and beauty and supported artisans from all around the world. And as I reach further back, I see my grandmother Sheila who was a feminist and started a women's job-counseling center in the 1970s. My grandmothers Sheila and Milka, both of whom were a large presence in my life, passed away well into their late nineties within months of each other in the winter of 2016–2017. They couldn't have been more different in character, but they were both so fully themselves.

My grandmother Sheila was an avid gardener, sailor, and writer and a strong and fiercely independent woman. From a young age, I witnessed Sheila's reverence for plants and the tides. She spent every summer in the far northern town of Sorrento, Maine, where my father spent his childhood summers as well. He learned how to run through the forest barefoot, knowing every rock and root as I did. I would often spend weeks with her in her home there. She taught me how to tie knots and eat lettuce fresh from the garden (dirt and all), and she pushed me out to sea in a rowboat, telling me to row back to shore. Sheila was also always nose-deep in a book on a dizzying array of subjects. She loved to research and wrote several books on environmentalism, city planning, and our family history. She instilled in me a love of writing and research, even on obscure subjects. The wild landscape of Sorrento has remained one of the main poles of inspiration for my products. After Sheila passed away, I came into possession of the sailor's log she kept during the 1940s. Her droll humor, sarcastic laugh, and sharp wit resound in her descriptions of sails around Sorrento. Her writing exudes clear information and sage wisdom mixed with so much personality.

My grandmother Milka grew up in the mountains of Montenegro. She was an agricultural engineer, and my grandfather was a forestry engineer, and when my mother was growing up, the family split their time between Belgrade and a tiny rural Serbian town called Brusnik. From Serbia they moved to Morocco, where Milka studied cosmetology as a trade, and, among other things, she learned to use argan oil directly on her skin and hair. She taught me about the importance of self-care. I have so many memories of sitting on a stool by her knees as she would brush my hair. One of my last memories of Milka is of her brushing my daughter Mila's hair.

As a teenager, I spent a number of summers in Brusnik living in the old stone house, surrounded by orchards, that has been in our family for over five hundred years. Each morning, one of our neighbors would roll a watermelon from their fields to our door. Figs dripped from trees in the yard, and daily we feasted on the most delicious tomatoes, whose name in Serbo-Croatian is aptly *paradajz*. My grand-mother knew how to make fresh herbal tea. She drank brandy from the fruits of the land, and she knew how to care naturally for the body inside and out, with simple, fresh food and simple, fresh skincare.

As a mother, I wonder what lessons my two small children will gather over time from me. My daughter, Mila, likes to play Captain Blankenship, making pretend lip balms for herself and friends. My daughter and son, Caspian, learned to crawl amid packing supplies, boxes full of bottles, and vials of essential oils. I hope my children learn from me what I learned from my family: that you can move through the world with passion and creativity, striving to be fully yourself.

Captain Blankenship, my company, was born in 2009. I was working full-time but had been making products on the side for myself, family, and friends. Playing alchemist in my kitchen was where you would find me those days; or, for inspiration, hiking in the Berkeley hills, full of fragrant eucalyptus groves. It felt so satisfying and electric to be creating products that I believed in and that people enjoyed in their own rituals.

I began to study and understand the beautiful raw ingredients that came from plants and their many uses in self-care. It was exhilarating to be able to count the ingredients I put in my products on my hands and know exactly what they were, why they were there, and where they came from. My friends had started an incredible store called Gravel & Gold in San Francisco and wanted to start carrying some of the things I was creating. I figured I had better start a company. I went forward with no business plan, no capital beyond my savings account, no idea where it would go, but full of the passion to create.

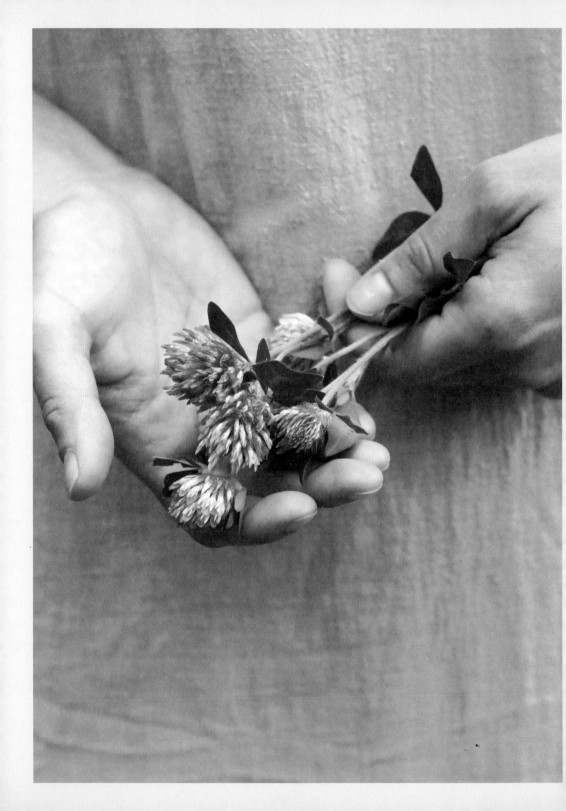

This desire to create products with integrity, and ones that affect people's lives, is both a joy and a privilege I don't take lightly. From my experiences, I have learned so much about the slippery category of beauty and its dangerous potential. Beauty tied to an ideal and sold with damaging chemicals is something that, in my opinion, stinks. I know that other people have caught the whiff as well; there is currently a sea change in the beauty world as both retailer and customer are embracing green products over their conventional rivals. What I seek to share in my products isn't the promise of the impossible; it's the intelligence of nature. I believe that these oils, butters, and extracts from plants and minerals can help make our skin, hair, body, and spirit healthier and more vibrant.

Our motto at Captain Blankenship is "Beauty Wild with Nature," which to me means you will find the beauty, wildness, and wisdom of the ocean, fields, and forests reflected in every bottle. I truly believe beauty is a process that is inextricably connected to your health, wellness, and state of mind. In this book, I've included the most important findings from my research and experimentation, my favorite ingredients, and the ones I think it is best to avoid. I've also shared anecdotes and tips with you, as well as simple recipes to promote healthy skin, hair, and well-being, helping you to radiate your beauty from the inside out. Anchors aweigh.

CHAPTER ONE

Trusting Your Nose

"Of all the senses, the sense of smell is the one that reaches most readily beyond us even as it most powerfully taps the wellsprings of our inmost selves. It has an unparalleled capacity to wake us up, to make us fully human."[2]

Mandy Aftel, *Fragrant*

*I*like to think my husband, Levi, and I moved to Berkeley because of the jasmine. Our first visit was in April, and the fragrance washed over everything, a bright watermelon haze tinged with narcotic floral waves. At the time, I had no idea that jasmine was one of my favorite smells, but walking by walls of jasmine vines immediately lifted my spirits. While I still relished the scents of the natural world, I mostly buried my nose for fear of a negative reaction from synthetic fragrance.

One day, I walked into a friend's store and smelled a solid perfume made from jasmine absolute, grapefruit, and blood orange essential oils, beautifully encased in a sterling silver compact. It smelled sweet and breathtaking, like the flowers and citrus growing in the hills outside. I bought it, wore it, and was smitten. I sought out the amazing perfumer who made it, Mandy Aftel, studied with her, and never looked back. The world of essential oils opened to me a rich and invisible palette more evocative than anything I had ever encountered.

Scent is one of the first senses to develop in the womb. When a baby meets its mother, it recognizes her by smell, and she recognizes the unique smell of her child. If you were to ask most people which sense they would first sacrifice, most people say smell. But if you lose your sense of smell, an affliction called *anosmia*, much of the pleasure is stripped from your life. Food doesn't taste good if you can't smell its aroma. The people you love lose dimension without their characteristic smells. Familiar things become dull without their signature scents.

Invisible pillars made of scent hold up the architecture of our individual and sometimes collective memories. Smells travel through our nostrils to our olfactory bulb, which links to two areas of our brain: the amygdala, which is tied to emotion, and the hippocampus, which is linked to memory. Knowing this, it makes complete sense that a smell can instantly beckon age-old memories or summon emotions in a whiff.

I once made a perfume called Phosphorescent. It was an intriguing mix of tangerine, honeysuckle, vanilla, and seaweed. To me, it conjured a summer day, the beach, sunscreen, and glowing phosphorescence in the ocean at night. Though it may sound odd, I thought of it as a briny Creamsicle. I recognize that the scent of seaweed is an acquired taste, but to me, it has always brought me back to the ocean, my constant source of inspiration and wonder.

I took an introduction to natural perfumery class with Mandy at the Esalen Institute and felt emboldened and inspired to start making my own blends. Mandy is a brilliant pioneer in the world of natural perfumery, and her deep passion and intimate knowledge of plant essences unlocked a world of wonder for me. Do yourself a big favor and pick up and plunge into her book *Essence and Alchemy* if you haven't read it yet. Esalen, the historic institute and retreat perched on cliffs above crashing waves in Big Sur, is the perfect place to let go and learn. Getting to know the oils—spending time smelling them, learning how they wear over time, getting a sense of their character—was like learning a new language. It was thrilling to experience them and still is.

Many years later, Mandy is my dear friend and mentor, whose kindness, generosity, wisdom, and support keep me diving deeper in my craft. It feels so right to me that she awoke my olfactory calling in Big Sur, surrounded by the wild coastline and crashing waves. To me, the landscape feels very kindred to the rocky shores of my Maine childhood. From that time on, I collected essential oils and made it my job to follow my nose and experiment with this new palette. I can't wait to take you on an adventure into the invisible and evocative world of plant essences.

The Heart of Plants

Essential oils are the most concentrated form of a plant's aroma. Made from the distilled roots, bark, leaves, seeds, and fruit of a plant, the oils are precious, powerful, and must be used wisely. With any artform, one must know the tools intimately to be able to experiment freely.

Mandy Aftel describes our relationship to aromas as "a magic carpet we can ride to hidden worlds, not only to other times and places but deep within ourselves, beneath the surface of daily life."[3] The perfumer's organ is the name of the cabinet or shelf that houses their precious collection of aromatic materials.

WATERY BEGINNINGS

"Our sense of smell, like so many body functions,
is a throwback to that time, early in evolution, when
we thrived in the oceans. An odor must first dissolve
into a watery solution our mucous membranes
absorb before we smell it."[4]

DIANE ACKERMAN

In her seminal book, *A Natural History of the Senses*, Diane Ackerman describes the prehistoric evolution of smell in our amphibian ancestors to help them find mates and avoid danger, tools that we could still harness with our noses. To think about scent evolving deep in the ocean was a revelation to me.

Ackerman describes an epiphany she had her first time scuba diving, "Scuba diving in the Bahamas some years ago, I became aware of two things for the first time: that we carry the ocean within us; that our veins mirror the tides . . . I was so moved, my eyes teared underwater, and I mixed my saltiness with the ocean's."[5]

Ackerman's realization resonates with every cell of my watery being. Some of my greatest moments of belonging were floating on a salty ocean, feeling rocked gently by the waves. Nature, which we sometimes regard as other, holds the secrets of our being. For me, the privilege of working with botanical scents is getting to relish in the beauty of plants and celebrate their power and medicine. Just as we evolved in the mother ocean, we must still look to nature to nourish and help us evolve.

From the organ, the perfumer can access and smell the best oils sourced from around the globe. I often am asked if I grow all my raw materials and make all my essential oils myself. I wish I lived on a lavender farm, but, alas, I don't. I prefer to source my oils from people whose families have been growing and distilling oils for decades, or even centuries, honoring and supporting their craft and their wisdom. The best organic rose essential oil I have smelled comes from Bulgaria, my favorite vetiver essential oil comes from Indonesia, and I think the most beautiful blood orange essential oil comes from Sicily.

The use of essential oils dates back to at least 3000 BCE. Egyptians prized essential oils for use in beauty rituals, medicinal preparations, and spiritual practices. Perhaps the most famous user of natural ingredients in the ancient world was Cleopatra, who used essential oils, carrier oils, natural clays, and Dead Sea salts in her beauty regimen. Essential oils were also used in India, China, and ancient Rome in daily life. In the Middle Ages, essential oils were prescribed to ward off the plague. Thieves who robbed the houses of those ill with the bubonic plague infamously developed the well-known remedy called Thieves Oil. Made of a potent mix of clove, cinnamon, eucalyptus, rosemary, and lemon essential oils, it literally was (and still is) used as a cloak to keep sickness at bay.

Essential oils are made through the steam distillation of plant material. Over the ages, many tools have been used to extract essential oils. The hand-hammered copper alembic still is the most iconic method of extraction, but there are also repurposed whisky stills and glass stills. The Latin term *per fumus* means "through smoke," revealing how material is heated to extract its precious essence. Steam distillation is a way of extracting the plant's vitality. The plant's volatile molecules are literally vaporized in steam and then cooled and reconstituted as oil. The process of steam distillation separates a plant's molecules from its cellulose, the organic polymer of plants. There is a lot of variation in the yield of essential oil from plant to plant, but generally, it ranges from 1 percent to 10 percent oil per distillation.

As you may know from buying essential oils, a small vial can be incredibly expensive. There can be anywhere between several pounds and hundreds of thousands of pounds of plant material in the still, so you can get a sense of how valuable plant essences can be. It takes 60,000 pounds of rose petals to make 1 pound of precious oil. In most cases, a few drops go a long way.

Different essential oils have varying scent intensities. For instance, a powerful scent such as basil can quickly swallow a delicate scent such as neroli. When creating a blend, it is always best to proceed with caution. Start with fewer drops and slowly increase; you can always add, but you can't subtract.

Hydrosols

Have you ever used rosewater on your skin or in cooking? It is one of my favorites to refresh, both for my skin and to drink. Rosewater is an aromatic hydrosol, which is a by-product of steam distillation. When you distill plant material to make essential oils, you are left with oil floating on top of water. The essential oils are separated out, and the leftover water is beautifully infused with the plant essence. Hydrosols are a perfect union of water and plants. They can be used for any number of things, including face and body mists or as a base for lotions or creams. In addition, many can also be ingested. Imagine, the public baths in Ancient Rome were filled with rosewater as places to relax, revive, and indulge the senses.

While rosewater is a popular hydrosol, through steam distillation a hydrosol can be made from almost any plant. Even flowers such as jasmine, which will not produce essential oils, can be made into a beautiful scented hydrosol. Lavender and orange blossom are also popular. The one thing about hydrosols is that they are volatile. Each hydrosol has a different shelf life, so it is safest to keep them in the refrigerator to keep them stable. Nothing is more refreshing than spritzing a cold hydrosol on your face on a hot day.

Scent Extractions

Lilac is one of those scents that transports me right back to childhood. There was a huge purple bush in our backyard. When it bloomed, I would put my face in it, close my eyes, and inhale the sweet, green scent. Unfortunately, the climate in the Bay Area doesn't nurture lilacs along with the amazing flora that thrive there. I forgot when I lived out there how short a window lilacs have for blooming. Now living in New York, I have planted many bushes side by side to create the fragrant lilac wall of my dreams. I await the arrival of mid-May each year and the first blossoms on the bush, but it always comes and goes way too quickly. The longing just makes the experience all the more precious.

However, many exquisite but delicate flowers such as lilac, jasmine, lotus, orange blossom, tuberose, magnolia, frangipani, and violet leaf cannot be distilled into essential oils. As soon as you heat them in a still, their stunning scent evaporates without a trace. Luckily, there are other processes to extract their beautiful essence.

ENFLEURAGE

Enfleurage is a process developed in eighteenth-century France that uses fats such as lard or tallow that are solid at room temperature to extract odor molecules from plants. Plant materials such as jasmine blossoms are added to the fat, and over time, they infuse the fat with their essence. The blossoms are replaced by new ones, and the process is repeated until the desired fragrance

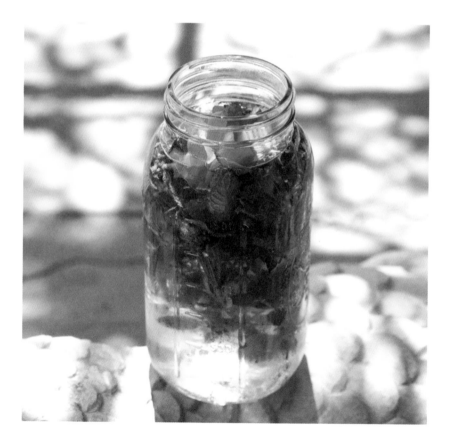

saturation is achieved. The scented fat can be used as pomade or it can be soaked into ethyl alcohol to draw out the odor molecules into a solvent. This process is romantic but inefficient and rarely used anymore.

CONCRETES

To make a concrete, plant materials, usually flowers, are covered with a solvent, usually hexane, which is used to dissolve the essential oils. Through this process, the flowers create a soft wax that collects the oils, which is called a concrete. Concretes are semisolid and not fully dissolvable in alcohol. They were traditionally used to scent soaps but are not commonly used anymore.

ABSOLUTE

The absolute is the most expensive and longest-wearing type of extract in natural perfumery. To make an absolute, the concrete is dissolved into ethanol. (Some people prefer not to use concretes and absolutes due to the solvent extraction process.) You can definitely smell the difference between an essential oil and an absolute. My favorite comparison for this is lavender. Lavender essential oil smells very different depending on the grade you use, but it most often smells antiseptic, floral, and sharp. Lavender absolute has an altogether different scent; it is very fresh and green, like actual lavender blossoms pressed between your fingers.

CO_2 EXTRACT

A CO_2 (carbon dioxide) extraction is a relatively modern innovation that has gained popularity in the past fifty years. CO_2 is a supercritical fluid, meaning it converts to liquid when placed under extreme pressure. By utilizing changes in pressure, CO_2 extraction removes essential oils from plant matter without leaving any solvent residue behind. This process is also gentler than the other distillation techniques and is popular for cannabis oil extraction.

ISOLATES

In contrast to a whole essential oil found in a plant, isolates are single-odor molecules that are physically isolated or separated from natural compounds. A natural isolate is a molecule that is isolated from a plant, such as rose or mint. These isolates are a fraction of an essential oil. Isolated aromatics do not smell like the plant they are derived from and can expand the perfumer's palette in unique ways. For example, alpha ionone derived from the citrusy *Litsea cubeba* essential oil smells like freshly picked violets. Natural isolates are derived from plants, unlike those produced by various laboratory processes, such as synthetic biology, in which isolates are synthesized using bacteria and fungi.

SYNTHETIC FRAGRANCES

The specter of natural perfumery is synthetic fragrance. Synthetic fragrances were first introduced in Europe in the mid-1800s, when scientists learned how to isolate single-odor molecules from plant material. Natural isolates are the constituents of an essential oil. Maybe you have seen linalool, geraniol, limonene, or citronellol on ingredient lists; these are natural isolates. An essential oil is a reflection of the properties of the whole plant. An isolate is a constituent of the oil removed from the plant to capture its scent or properties. It wasn't long after scientists learned how to isolate odor molecules that they learned how to synthesize them. Synthetic fragrances are designed in a laboratory to mimic and expand upon the scents of the natural world. Coumarin, the first synthetic note to enter perfumery, was developed by British chemist William Henry Perkin in 1868. Perkin derived coumarin from compounds found in coal tar, but coumarin is also found naturally in sources such as tonka beans and cinnamon. In my humble opinion, this bout of alchemy is incredible but also pretty unappealing. The scent of coumarin is said to smell like fresh hay and is a widely used fixative in modern perfumery. Synthetic replicas for scents grew with increasing demand because they were cheap and readily available.[6]

Synthetics were fashionable and initially integrated with essential oils in perfume blends such as Jicky Guerlain, a wildly popular fragrance for women created in 1889. Then synthetics took over the industry, which didn't look back, as evidenced by the groundbreaking Chanel No. 5. These new scents were called "modern" as opposed to "natural." Instead of being harvested from the field and manifested into oils of rich hues, these oils were colorless substances manufactured in a lab. Currently, one of the biggest fragrance houses in the world is International Flavors and Fragrances. It developed the proprietary synthetic scents that fragrance such things as perfumes, deodorants, and laundry detergents, and it also developed such flavors as the newest taste trend in potato chips. Scents are proprietary, and in the United States, personal care and perfume companies do not have to disclose the hundreds or even thousands of unregulated chemicals that comprise their recipes; they are classified as "trade secrets." They are hidden away in the word *fragrance* or *parfum* on their ingredient lists. As harmless as these words sound, little do most consumers know the Pandora's box that lies within.

The term *natural fragrance* indicates that the scent in a product is made from a blend of isolates. This means the manufacturer is not using whole essential oils but using isolates extracted from them to create a scent not found in nature. You better believe that if a company is using only essential oils to scent its products instead of synthetics, it will wear this information proudly on its packaging and in its ingredient lists.

The scent of something as ubiquitous as Old Spice or Tide detergent comes from a synthetic chemical cocktail. These scents meant to freshen actually stay on our clothes and our skin and can even enter our bloodstreams. Many perfumers who claim their scents are natural often add synthetics in small doses to increase their duration. If it is important to you to wear only plant-based essences, always read the ingredients closely. Synthetic fragrance can be hiding in places you don't suspect.

Later I will detail a list of some of the synthetic fragrance ingredients to avoid, but the potential negative effects range from migraines to skin irritation to severe respiratory reactions. Some of these ingredients have been classified as endocrine disrupters; they may be carcinogenic and have been linked to both neurotoxicity and birth defects.

When I smell a synthetic fragrance, it summons nothing of the natural world to me. It smells one-dimensional and aggressive. Synthetic scents are cloying, sticking to everything they touch, which to some people is comforting. The scent of the laundry detergent or soap that you have always used conjures stability and positive feelings. People value fragrance oils for their long-lasting wear, and they can become a continuous cloak of confidence. I, on the other hand, am fond of the ephemerality and vulnerability of essential oil–based scents. Like the waning of the day, they fade and evolve over time. Instead of a static scent, they transform and react. It is a matter of preference, but as people become more and more sensitive to synthetic chemicals, it is also a matter of clearing the air.

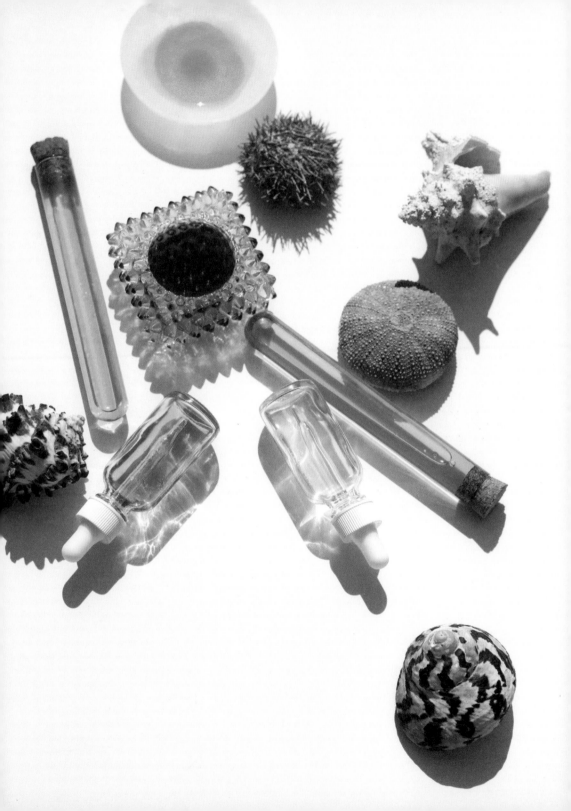

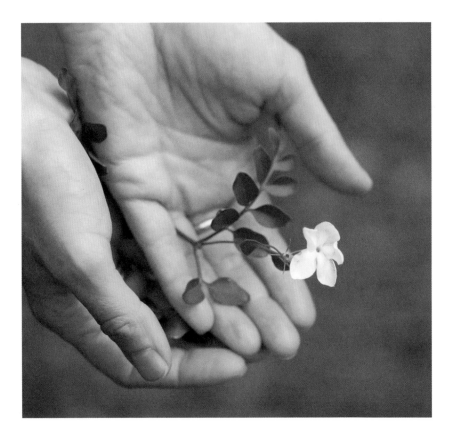

As we start to lose touch with the scents of the natural world, we lose touch with a primal part of ourselves. I believe we need to reclaim our noses and reconnect to the scents of the natural world. When we breathe, we smell. Inhaling is a part of our vitality and a vibrant practice for well-being.

Carriers

Carriers, either plant-based oils or alcohol, transport essential oils and aromatics to the skin. In aromatherapy or face and body oils, oils such as jojoba, sunflower seed, or rosehip seed can act as a base to blend with essential oils or extracts. You can choose a carrier oil or mix of oils based on what your skin needs. For an aromatherapy blend, jojoba or safflower oils are good as they don't have a heavy scent to interfere with the strength of the essential oils, and they are easily absorbed. For a face oil or body oil, you can tailor the carrier oils to your skin's needs.

I like to use both alcohol and oil as carriers for a perfume or aromatherapy blend, depending on the situation. Alcohol provides a lighter feel on skin and a complex fragrance. If I am making a spray perfume, I always go with alcohol. I like to use organic grape or sugarcane alcohol, but any high-proof neutral grain spirit can work.

Oil-based perfumes are thicker and more concentrated, but they tend to have a subtler and softer aroma than alcohol-based scents, which come on strong but will evaporate more quickly. Choose a carrier oil with a long shelf life that has little scent of its own. I prefer to use jojoba oil since it is the closest oil to our own sebum, and it doesn't have much of a smell. If I am making a roll-on perfume, I tend to choose oil as a base.

Aromatherapy

Aromatherapy is a word that is thrown around a lot these days, but we only need to look to the word itself to get a general idea of its meaning. Aromatherapy means therapy through scent, and harnessing the power of scent as a conscious tool can lead to healing physically, emotionally, and spiritually.

Aromatherapy is an ancient art, but it was formally named by chemist René-Maurice Gattefossé in 1920s France. His first book was titled *Aromathérapie,* and the rest is history. Part of the impetus for his exploration in aromatherapy was the result of a chemical explosion in his lab that left his hand seriously burned.[7] He instinctually dipped his hand in lavender essential oil and found that through repeated application, his hand healed within days. This propelled him research the healing power of plants, which grew into the modern-day practice of aromatherapy.

THROUGH SMOKE

The Latin root of perfume, meaning "through smoke," underscores how perfumes were used through the ages. The rituals of lighting incense or candles and smudging (burning sacred herbs) are all ancient practices that represent a connection with something larger. By letting smoke rise up to the sky, we activate and transform space as well as honor our ancestors and ourselves.

A ROSE IS A ROSE ISN'T A ROSE

The word *chemical* is thrown around these days as the opposite of the words *natural* and *organic*. Yet, we are made of chemicals, as is the air we breathe. There are ninety-two naturally occurring chemical elements on Earth.

Rachel Herz, a psychologist and a cognitive neuroscientist as well as an expert on the psychology of smell, reveals some interesting perceptions about natural versus synthetic fragrance.

"Smells are chemicals, and they can be extremely complex and contain thousands of molecules, like the rose scent emanating from your flower bed, which is made up of between twelve hundred and fifteen hundred different molecules. Or they can be very simple and comprise just one molecule, like phenylethyl alcohol, the chemical that imparts the scent of rose in many commercial hand lotions."[8]

The true scent of a rose is much more complex and many-layered as compared with the one-dimensional fake rose scent. The rose in your garden could be one of thousands of varieties, and it could smell like tea, sweet, warm, floral, spicy, or any number of other adjectives. Yet, as our noses become more accustomed to the ubiquitous fake rose scents, we are losing our grasp on real smells.

One of my favorite scents in the world is the sweet and spicy scent of the *Rosa rugosa*. For me, the smell conjures the beach in Maine in the summer, where thorny hot-pink roses with deep green foliage spread along the edges of the shore. I have a precious vial of this essential oil that I reach for when I am down. My scent memory is so deeply infused with this smell that no synthetic scent could fool me. I truly hope!

Incense has played a role in all cultures since ancient times. Traditionally, incense was made of natural materials such as wood, leaves, needles, flowers, herbs, and spices that are ground up together and reconstituted into cones or sticks. These materials conjure the forest and field, yet they gain another dimension entirely when they turn to smoke. Nag champa incense, traditionally made from a combination of pure sandalwood and the fragrant frangipani flower, has been used to scent monasteries in India for centuries. Many modern-day versions of this ancient incense are made using synthetic fragrance oils, which are anything but subtle.

Frankincense and myrrh are both made from the oozing sap of trees when their bark is cut. They have been used in ceremony and personal care for at least five thousand years. Frankincense comes from the Boswellia tree, and myrrh from the Commiphora tree. Resin-like in texture, they produce a very sweet, piney, citrus scent when burned together. Ancient Egyptians used this heady combination as incense, perfumes, and salves. Ancient Greeks, Romans, Jews, and Christians burned them in sacred rituals. Their popularity made these saps worth their weight in gold, and they continue to be used ceremonially, in perfumes, and in personal preparations for their healing properties.

Many Native American tribes use the ceremony of smudging as a practice of spiritual cleansing and blessing. Traditionally, white sage and red cedar are bound together into a smudge stick, which is lit, and the smoke is used to clear negative energy.

Palo santo means "holy wood" in Spanish. The palo santo tree belongs to the Burseraceae family, a relative of frankincense, myrrh, and copal. Fallen branches and twigs of the tree have been used in South America dating back to the Incas, for ceremonial purposes. Palo santo is used in much the same way as smudging to clear negative energy.

Ancient Egyptians are credited with developing the first candles in 3000 BCE by dipping reeds in animal fat. It was the Romans who created the first wicked candles and started using beeswax as a base. Candles, of course, have always been used as an important source of light, but they've also been used as connection to something larger in personal and communal rituals.

ALTERNATIVES TO FIRE

I used to love smudging my home until I had small children. The smoke was too heavy for them, so I created a smokeless smudge spray with white sage and other powerful essential oils to achieve a similar cleansing effect. I love to smudge my home, but I like to alternate with the spray. You can also use an essential oil diffuser as an effective way to gently fill a space with scent.

Primal Magic

When I first started experimenting with natural perfumery, I had recently adopted a Siberian husky puppy that we named Vuka, which means wolf. Dogs have an incredibly keen sense of smell, and I always wondered what she must think of the strange scent experiments I was making in our house; was it pleasant, alarming, or both? The answer is most likely neither. A dog's sense of smell is radically different from our own; they possess 300 million olfactory receptors in their noses, while we only have a pithy 6 million. To Vuka, her nose is an integral tool. While we primarily identify the people we know by sight, she smells them coming. When a dog raises its nose in the air, she is gathering information. When she marks a spot, she is starting a conversation that another dog might add to. She can sense emotion, fear, illness, or age in body odor, death, urine, and feces. She knows my smell intimately; she smells it in my footprints, which is how she finds me in the forest.[9]

Think about the importance of smell as our own unique way of identifying ourselves. Then think of a wall of conventional deodorants and perfumes; the two are at odds. I dream of the day Glade PlugIns and those Christmas-tree air fresheners will be black-market items. I actually don't think it is that far off. Many private spaces such as yoga studios limit fragrance, and as people become more sensitive to synthetics, it is a matter of time before the lawsuits start.

Call me a purist, but I think things should smell good naturally, including you. Enhancing scent naturally is one thing, but masking it entirely is a crime. So, instead of cloying scents, let's make some magic that will spark emotions and memories and will gently fade over time.

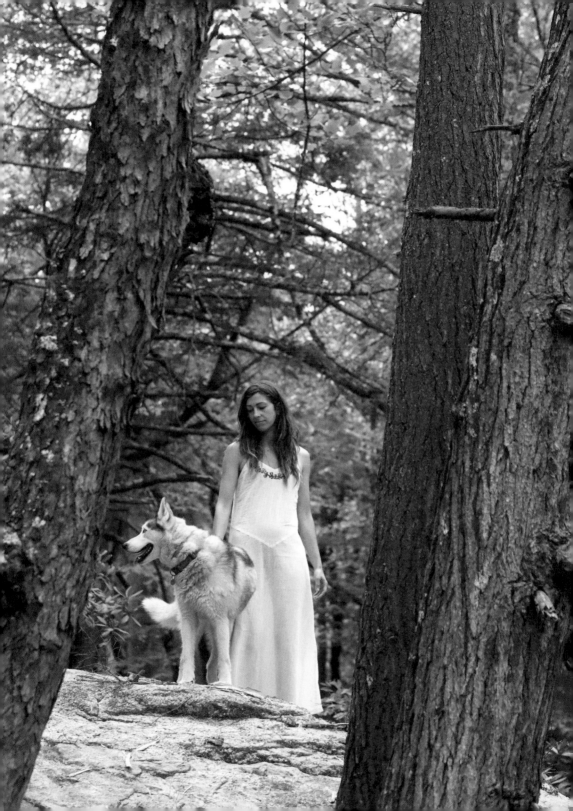

CHAPTER TWO

Aromatics

"Follow your heart like a nose follows smell."[10]

Maria Soledad, in conversation with author

*I*magine you could dive into a bottle of natural perfume and inspect and savor every ingredient and each distinct smell. The perfumer creates work that is more than a sum of its parts, like an alchemist who transmutes matter into spirit. Perfume reacts differently on each body it touches because everyone's body chemistry and sense of smell are different. In addition, each plant essence has its own structure that, when combined into a perfume, becomes something else entirely, a harmonious work of art. A perfume is traditionally made of base notes, middle notes, and top notes, which is a direct reference to music. When certain scents align and enhance each other, they are called *chords*. To create a well-balanced perfume is to develop a real harmony, one in which each element depends on the others to make it sing. Let's delve into how we grow a harmonious perfume from the ground up.

In a simple blend, you could choose one base note, one middle note, and one top note to start. In more complicated perfumes, you could have three or four of each note. Before diving in, it is helpful to take some time to reflect on the character of the perfume you want to create. If you want orange blossom to be a star in your perfume, you should try not to bury it with heavier scents. Take some time to brainstorm before you start blending. You can always add more drops, but you cannot subtract them. There is nothing sadder than creating mud out of precious materials and needing to start over.

In this chapter, I want to introduce you to some of my favorite essential oils and then some simple recipes for scent blends for well-being, room sprays, and perfumes. That said, scent is entirely subjective, and you may have different preferences than I do. Feel free to adjust the scent blends to your liking, and above all, trust your nose. You are the most important ingredient.

Base Notes

Mandy Aftel uses the metaphor of a tree to talk about plant essences. The base notes are the roots of the tree, the resinous scents that build the foundation of a perfume. They often are made from actual roots, like vetiver. Other popular base notes include frankincense, myrrh, vanilla, patchouli, palo santo, sandalwood, seaweed, oak moss, and violet leaf. These base notes are heavy, rich, and syrupy in smell and are what gives perfume longevity. When building a perfume, you work from the ground up.

WOODS, ROOTS & RESINS

Myrrh (*Commiphora myrrha*) is the resin from the Commiphora shrub that has been used for ritual and healing purposes since ancient times. You might also find it in your toothpaste, as it is powerful for gum infections and gingivitis. It is wonderful for very dry and cracked skin, hands and feet, and skin conditions such as eczema. In perfume, it adds a velvety warmth and richness.

Frankincense (*Boswellia carterii*) comes from a shrub-like tree and has been used for healing, rejuvenative, and aromatherapeutic purposes since ancient times. Frankincense and myrrh go hand in hand in a powerful incense used for spiritual purposes. An essential oil and absolute are made from the gum resin of the tree. Frankincense smells fresh, rich, woody, and ethereal. It is great for all skin types and for wound healing. It also helps ease stress and anxiety and improves focus, making it a powerful aid for meditation.

Patchouli (*Pogostemon cablin*) is a bushy herb whose leaves are made into the ubiquitous spicy and earthy essential oil. Many people instantly write off patchouli as a strong aroma used to cover up pot smoke, but it is an essential oil with a lot of depth. Aged patchouli has a rich, syrupy, smoky scent, like a peaty Scotch.

Sandalwood (*Santalum album, spicatum, paniculatum,* or *Eucarya spicata*) is the prized essential oil made from the distilled wood of the aromatic sandalwood tree. It is one of the oldest and most distinctive-smelling materials in perfumery, and the wood is also used as a sacred building material. Several varieties of sandalwood are native to Australia, Southeast Asia, Indonesia, Sri Lanka, Taiwan, India, and Hawaii. Because of the high demand for the essential oil, concern has been raised over the sustainability of sandalwood production resulting from deforestation in native habitats. If you purchase sandalwood essential oil, make sure that it has been sustainably harvested. The tree must be at least thirty years old to be ready for essential oil production, which makes it incredibly precious. The scent of the oil smells like sandalwood shavings: rich, woody, and sweet. Dried and powdered, it is made into incense for spiritual rituals. Sandalwood oil is great for all skin types and as an aid for nerves, stress, and depression.

Vanilla (*Vanilla planifolia*) is the prized extract that comes from a vanilla pod or bean. Used widely as a flavoring and fragrance ingredient, vanilla adds a rich, sweet, and syrupy touch to perfumes. There is no essential oil made from vanilla, but it is available as both a CO_2 extract and an absolute.

Vetiver (*Vetiveria zizanioides*) oil is one of my all-time favorites. It is grounding, smoky, and earthy; a thick, fresh, and wild scent made of the distilled roots of vetiver grass that grows alongside volcanoes. It is highly relaxing and helps with nerves, depression, and anxiety. It is great for oily skin, acne, and stiffness, aches, and pains. A great addition to a room spray, body oil, or bath salt recipe.

Middle Notes

From the roots, we come to the flowers and leaves of the tree: the middle notes, which are the precious heart of a scent. Flowers such as jasmine, rose, tuberose, ylang ylang, geranium, and orange blossom are middle notes. Leaves, needles, and grasses are also in this category, including eucalyptus, pine, spruce, cypress, and palmarosa.

FLOWERS

Jasmine (*Jasminum grandiflorum, sambac*) may be the most exquisite scent, but it is an acquired taste. Extremely sweet, rich, and floral, it also has what some might describe as fecal undertones. I am a lover of jasmine, and it is one of my favorite middle notes to add to perfumes. There are two species that are readily available as plant essences. The most common jasmine is the one of my dreams and memories, *Jasminum grandiflorum*. It is available as an absolute and CO_2 extract. *Jasminum sambac*, also known as Arabian jasmine, is less sweet and a little spicier but not as prevalent. Use jasmine to create a deeply floral heart in your perfume. It blends well with citrus, pine, fir needle, ylang ylang, patchouli, vetiver, vanilla, and sandalwood. Jasmine is also great in skin and body care, especially for dry and mature skin. This is precious stuff, and a few drops bring a bouquet of beauty.

Roman chamomile (*Anthemis nobilis*) flowers exude peaceful feelings. The relaxing, herbal, and fruity scent of chamomile is used to relax and calm in both perfumery and personal care. Much as chamomile tea is used to calm adults, promote sleep, and soothe colicky infants, it has similar uses in perfumery and aromatherapy. It is available in different varieties such as German chamomile, which has azulene as a constituent, an anti-inflammatory that is blue in hue. It lends a beautiful color to face oils, body oils, and perfumes.

Geranium and rose geranium (*Pelargonium graveolens*) oil is made from the distilled leaves, stalk, and pink flowers of the aromatic shrub. The scent of geranium is sharp, floral, and green but not too sweet. Both a stimulant and an antidepressant, geranium works wonders in aromatherapy for stress and anxiety and is also a mood booster. Perfect for all skin types, it is anti-inflammatory and astringent. Geranium works well in toners, face oils, and body oils. It is a great oil for keeping away ticks, especially when used in conjunction with peppermint. This combo is also great for hair and scalp oil since both oils help strengthen and stimulate hair growth.

Lavender (*Lavandula angustifolia, officinalis,* or *vera*) is iconic and active. Lavender not only possesses a powerful floral scent, but it is a natural antiseptic and sedative. It is also an abundant crop and thus a very economical oil to buy. Lavender is a very polarizing scent; some people find it cloying while some adore it. There are many different types of lavender essential oils, and each possesses a distinct scent depending on where the plant was grown. Lavender is farmed and grown from Oregon to New York to Bulgaria, as well as in France, Italy, and the other Mediterranean countries. The main type of lavender used to make essential oil is *Lavandula angustifolia,* also called *Lavandula officinalis* and *Lavandula vera,* but depending on the terroir it is grown in, the scent can vary heavily. Lavender has a wide variety of uses. In aromatherapy, it is used to calm and relax the body and mind, and it also has antiseptic properties to help heal wounds and bruises as well as soothe burns.

Lavandin (*Lavandula x intermedia*) is a hybrid lavender that has a higher yield of essential oils than other types of lavender and thus is usually less expensive. It has a higher camphor content, making its smell stronger and more medicinal and also unsuitable to treat burns. Lavender absolute, by contrast, is deep green and smells sweet, sharp, and floral, with no medicinal undertones.

Orange blossom and neroli (*Citrus aurantium* var. *amara*) are two different expressions of the intoxicating, fragrant blossoms of the bitter orange tree. Orange blossom

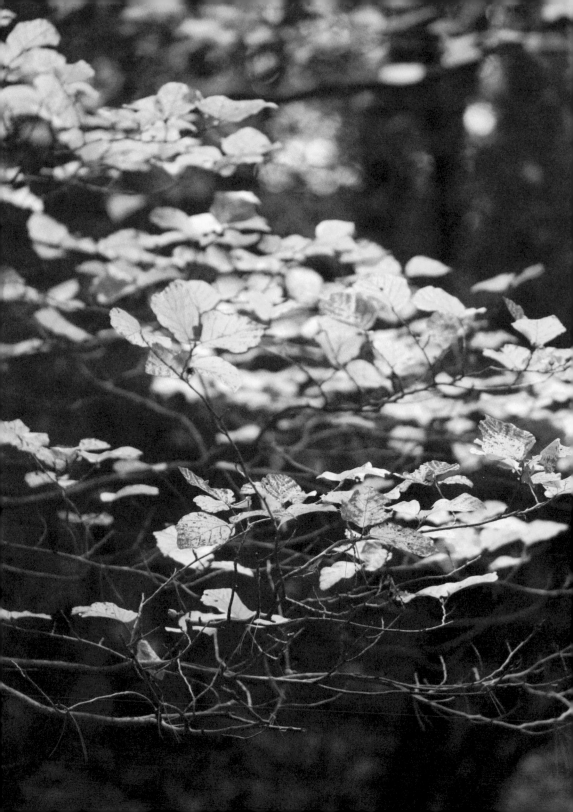

is a heavier, rich, syrupy citrus scent, reminiscent of plunging your nose into the delicate white blooms on an orange tree. It is made into both a CO_2 extract and an absolute. Neroli is the lighter of the two, more like the scent of orange blossoms floating on a breeze. Uplifting and fresh, neroli is made into an exquisite essential oil. It is a gorgeous addition to a perfume and, in aromatherapy, is powerful for treating anxiety, depression, and stress. Neroli is also great for dry and sensitive skin and is a delight in a face oil or toner.

Rose (*Rosa damascena, centifolia, rugosa, or odorata*) is the ancient flower queen whose petals scented fountains in Rome and perfumed Cleopatra's skin and hair. Floral, rich, spicy, sweet, delicate, airy, warm, sexy; there are as many adjectives to describe the smells of a rose as there are different varieties of the flower. The most common ones that are made into essential oils, CO_2 extracts, and absolutes are rose otto (*Rosa damascena*) and rose de mai (*Rosa centifolia*). Two other favorite varieties I treasure are the Chinese rose (*Rosa rugosa*) and tea rose (*Rosa odorata*). The scent of rose is beautiful, uplifting, and very powerful for working with grief and depression. Rose is also great for dry skin and hair, making it a wonderful addition to face, body, and hair oils. It is incredibly refreshing and hydrating in a toner or body mist. The essential oil and CO_2 extracts tend to be much more delicate in scent than the absolute. Rose is a precious and expensive ingredient, but a few drops can make a powerful potion.

Ylang ylang (*Cananga odorata*) is the sweet, floral, and slightly balsamic essential oil made from the yellow flowers of the tropical tree. Ylang ylang is an exquisite aphrodisiac and antidepressant and an inexpensive floral to use in perfumery. It is great for acne, eczema, rashes, inflammation, and hair and scalp health. A perfect addition to hair oil or scalp treatment, as the oil stimulates hair growth. There are several grades of ylang ylang oil, with subtle differences in scent. The first distillate that makes up 40 percent of oil production is ylang ylang extra. It is the most prized and the richest and creamiest scent. After that comes ylang ylang 1, 2, and 3, each subsequently less rich in smell.

LEAVES

Clary sage (*Salvia sclarea*) is not to be confused with common garden sage. It smells very different and much subtler. It is an exquisite oil with fresh, herbaceous, and slightly bitter green tea–like notes. Clary sage is great for acne, dandruff, and balancing oily skin and hair. An important oil for women's health, it is one of the most powerful oils for balancing hormones and relieving menstrual pain and hot flashes. It can be added to aromatherapy blends or used in a massage oil. This uplifting scent, with a dreamy quality that helps with depression and nerves, is also a natural aphrodisiac.

Eucalyptus (*Eucalyptus globulus*) smells like a grove of eucalyptus trees in the sun. Fresh and woody with a strong camphor smell, it is a powerful oil that can be used effectively in small doses. It is great for easing colds in a chest rub or bath, in a natural deodorant, or in aromatherapy blends for headaches. It can also help with circulation, aches, and pains, and is great in massage oil. The scent intensity is high, so use sparingly.

Fir (*Abies alba*) smells like a coniferous forest: green, refreshing, and invigorating. Fir essential oil is powerful for warding off colds and is a great ingredient in a winter bath salt or in a diffuser. It is one of my favorite smells, and I love adding it to products from massage oils to cleaning products. Since ancient Egyptian times, it has been used to promote hair growth and is perfect as part of a hair and scalp oil. There are several types of fir essential oils readily available, including silver fir, Douglas fir, Siberian fir, and, of course, holiday-superstar, balsam fir.

Juniper berry (*Juniperus communis*) is fresh, woody, and bright. The essential oil is distilled from the leaves and berries, emitting a scent like a breath of fresh air, adding a touch of the woods to perfume. It is great for oily skin and acne and as a toner and scalp treatment because of its astringent and antiseptic qualities. An effective addition to cold, flu, stress, and anxiety blends.

Pine (*Pinus sylvestris*) is made from the green needles of the proud pine tree. Green, woody, and fresh, it recalls a walk in a pine forest. It is a wonderful addition to a massage oil to help aches and pains and aid circulation. In the winter, it helps with colds, flu, and respiratory issues. Pine needle syrup is commonly used in cough and cold remedies as it is a natural expectorant with antimicrobial, antiviral, and antiseptic qualities. Pine essential oil is the perfect addition to a winter bath.

Tea tree (*Melaleuca alternifolia*) is a natural antiseptic and fungicide that is a part of nature's first-aid kit along with lavender. It can be used directly on skin and applied to wounds, burns, and insect bites. It is a well-known spot treatment for acne. It has a very heavy turpentine-like medicinal scent, which is too much for many people. You can dilute accordingly.

Lemongrass (*Cymbopogon citratus, schoenanthus,* or *flexuosos*) is an aromatic grass that is used for its culinary, aromatherapeutic, and medicinal properties. It smells like a lemony breeze, bright, cheerful, and tart sweet. A natural insecticide, it is a great-smelling addition to bug spray. It is a refreshing face toner, and is particularly good for acne-prone skin. In addition, it is a natural antiperspirant and is effective in massage oil for helping with poor circulation and muscle aches. It also helps relieve headaches and anxiety. The antimicrobial, bactericidal, and antiseptic properties of lemongrass make it a good addition to sanitizing and cleaning products.

Top Notes

The first wave of a perfume that you smell are the top notes, but they are fleeting. The top notes, the fruits of the tree, also include spices and herbs. All citrus fruits, spices, and most herbs are classified as top notes.

FRUIT

Citrus oils include white and ruby red grapefruit, bergamot, sweet orange, blood orange, tangerine, clementine, lemon, lime, and yuzu. Citrus is a definite mood booster and clarifying oil. Citrus oils in general are great for oily skin, acne, colds, infections, and mood boosting. These oils are phototoxic, so it is best not to use them on your skin before heading out into the sun.

HERBS

Peppermint and spearmint (*Mentha piperita* and *Mentha spicata*) will clear and stimulate your senses. A sniff is the perfect remedy for a headache or tiredness. They are refreshing, clearing, and mood boosting. Peppermint and spearmint share similar properties for aromatherapy and external uses, but spearmint is both gentler smelling and acting. Peppermint essential oil is also an insecticide and is great added to bug spray.

Diluted mint essential oils are also great for skin and hair. Mint is a wonderful addition to a refreshing toner or a clarifying hair and scalp rinse. It can tingle, so be careful to dilute before applying to skin and hair. If you get it directly on your nose or in your eyes, wash with lukewarm water and soap.

Basil and tulsi (*Ocimum basilicum, sanctum*) oils are bold, green, and anise-like, adding an herbal twist to any scent blend and helping with awakening your mind and opening your heart. The tulsi (holy basil) essential oil comes from the sweet, green, and woody basil that is native to India. It is popularly used in ayurveda, especially to support the third eye, our chakra of intuition.

Verbena or lemon verbena (*Lippia citriodora*) essential oil is a bold, delicious delight for the senses. Syrupy, sweet, green, and lemony, verbena helps boost your mood or brighten any scent.

Black Pepper (*Piper nigrum*) is a punctuation point in a perfume. Sharp, warm, and peppery, it dashes to the front door of a perfume and lets you in. It also blends beautifully with citrus. The pink peppercorn (*Schinus molle*) essential oil shares similar properties with black pepper, but it is softer and surprisingly floral.

Essential Oils During Pregnancy

Controversy abounds about which essential oils should not be used during pregnancy. Our sense of smell becomes heightened during pregnancy as a protective measure. I trust you to follow your nose. During my pregnancy with my daughter, Mila, I could not stand the smell of cedarwood and lavender, so I steered clear. Here is a general list of oils it is best to avoid since they can cause contractions or be unsafe for the mother or fetus:

OILS TO AVOID DURING PREGNANCY

ANISEED	DEERTONGUE	ROSEMARY
BASIL	FENNEL	RUE
BIRCH	HYSSOP	SAGE
CAMPHOR	JUNIPER BERRY	SASSAFRAS
CARAWAY	MARJORAM	TANSY
CASSIA	MUGWORT	TARRAGON
CEDARWOOD / THUJA	NUTMEG	TONKA
CINNAMON	OREGANO	WINTERGREEN
CLARY SAGE	PARSLEY	WORMWOOD
CLOVE	PENNYROYAL	

It is best to be cautious in the first trimester of pregnancy. If you use essential oils in your rituals, make sure that they are diluted. As always, follow your nose and stay away from things that don't smell good to you. Here is a list of essential oils that are safe to use in the second or third trimesters:

OILS THAT ARE SAFE DURING PREGNANCY

BERGAMOT	LEMON	ROMAN CHAMOMILE
EUCALYPTUS	LEMONGRASS	ROSE
FRANKINCENSE	LIME	ROSEWOOD
GERANIUM	MANDARIN	SANDALWOOD
GINGER	NEROLI	SWEET ORANGE
GRAPEFRUIT	PATCHOULI	TEA TREE
LAVENDER	PETITGRAIN	YLANG YLANG

A NOTE ON INGREDIENTS

I suggest using organic and wild-harvested essential oils, organic CO_2 extracts, and organic carrier oils, but you can experiment and see what you like best. As always, follow your nose.

Citrus essential oils should be kept in the fridge to keep them fresh. I like to use golden jojoba oil (not deodorized) for scent blends, but sunflower and safflower are also options. All three carrier oils are easily absorbed by the skin and don't carry much of a scent themselves, making them the perfect vehicle for essential oils.

A NOTE ON BLENDING

Please think of these as sketches that you can adapt to your liking. Scent is personal, and you should feel free to make changes and substitutions and make these your own work of art. Always remember you can add, but you can't subtract. Start slow with drops and add more if you desire. Cutting up scent strips made out of small strips of drawing paper and dipping them into your draft is a good way to get a sense of where the scent is and where you want to take it.

EQUIPMENT

Most of the equipment used in these recipes includes common kitchen items, such as a small pot, small strainer, mixing bowls, large and small heatproof spouted glass measuring cups, measuring spoons, metal spoons for stirring, spatula, and metal funnel. You will also need eyedroppers.

All of the ½-ounce recipes require glass aromatherapy roll-on bottles (use either a single ½-ounce bottle or two ¼-ounce bottles). All of the 4-ounce recipes require 4-ounce glass bottles with fine-mist sprayers. Additional items will be noted after the ingredient lists.

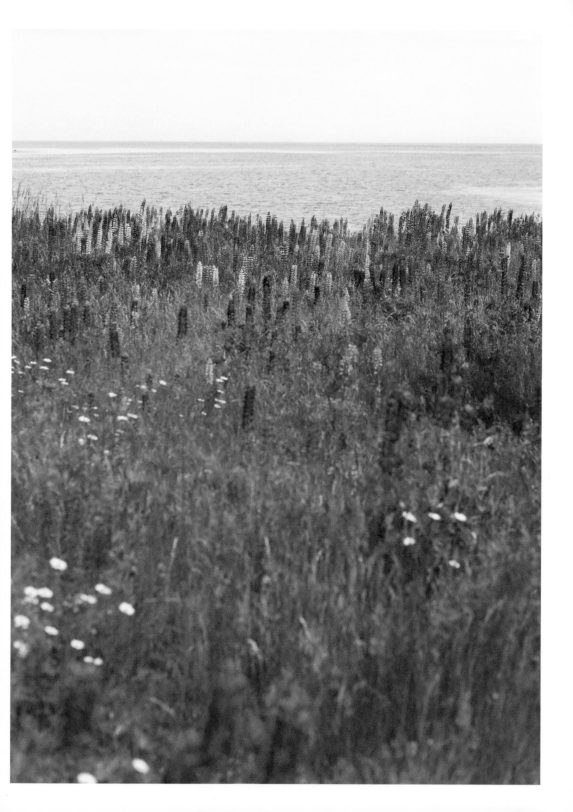

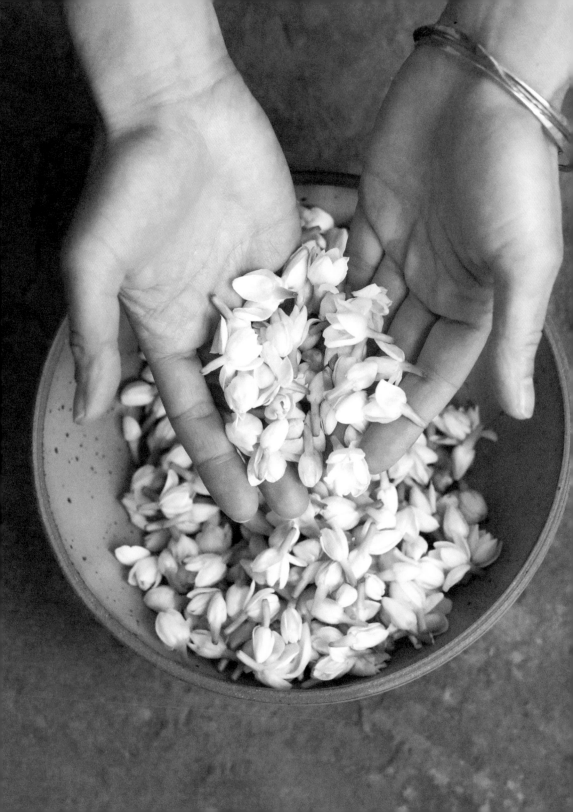

Vine Jasmine Blend

This blend mixes intoxicating jasmine with earthy vetiver, windy palmarosa, and juicy grapefruit to create a wild floral scent that captures the spirit of adventure. Dab it on your pulse points, behind your ears, or wherever you wish as often as you wish.

Add carrier oil to small spouted measuring cup. With separate eyedroppers, add essential oils to carrier oil and combine with a spoon. With funnel, pour slowly into roll-on bottles. Press on roll-on lid and screw on cap.

Use as needed. If stored out of direct sunlight, will keep for up to 2 years.

YIELD: ½ OUNCE

INGREDIENTS

1 tablespoon carrier oil of choice

8 drops grapefruit essential oil*
6 drops jasmine CO_2 extract
or absolute

5 drops palmarosa essential oil

3 drops vetiver essential oil

* I love pink and ruby red the best.

Vernal Neroli Blend

YIELD: ½ OUNCE

INGREDIENTS

1 tablespoon carrier oil of choice

7 drops neroli essential oil

6 drops fir balsam essential oil

6 drops frankincense essential oil

This simple but captivating trinity of neroli, fir balsam, and frankincense is ripe, ethereal, and green, like the coming of spring. Dab it on your pulse points or behind your ears.

Add carrier oil to small spouted measuring cup. With separate eyedroppers, add essential oils to carrier oil and combine with spoon. With funnel, pour slowly into roll-on bottles. Press on roll-on lid and screw on cap.

Use as needed. If stored out of direct sunlight, will keep for up to 2 years.

Venus Rose Blend

YIELD: ½ OUNCE

INGREDIENTS

1 tablespoon carrier oil of choice

7 drops sweet orange essential oil

6 drops rose essential oil

3 drops ylang ylang essential oil

3 drops vanilla CO_2 extract

This aphrodisiac blend smells like a warm rose in the sun. Rose, ylang ylang, sweet orange, and vanilla create a sweet, bright, and creamy scent with a hint of citrus sunlight. Dab it on your pulse points or behind your ears.

Add carrier oil to small spouted measuring cup. With separate eyedroppers, add essential oils to carrier oil and combine with spoon. With funnel, pour slowly into roll-on bottles. Press on roll-on lid and screw on cap.

Use as needed. If stored out of direct sunlight, will keep for up to 2 years.

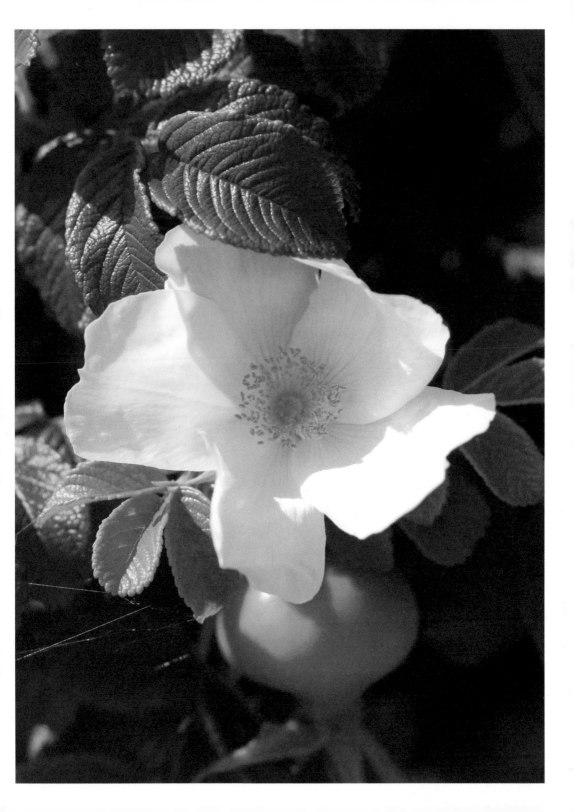

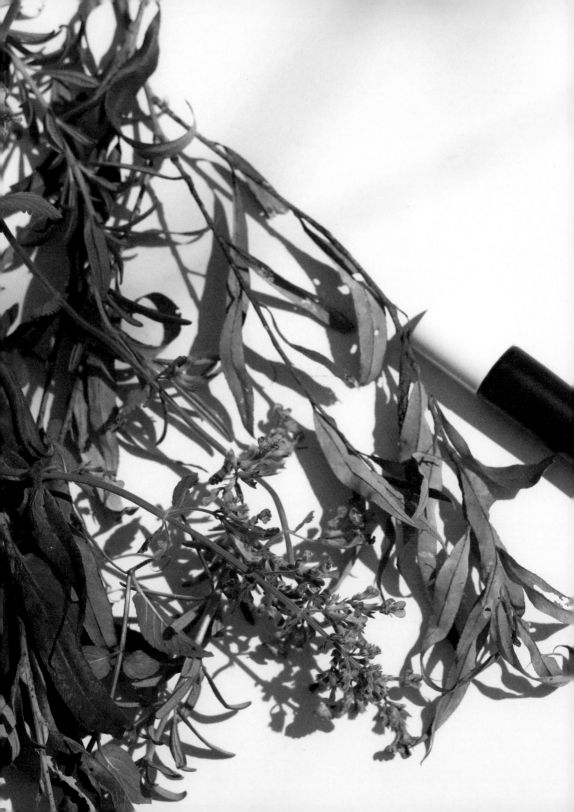

Loosen the Knot Tension-Release Blend

This powerful blend of essential oils is great for relieving anxiety, tension, headaches, migraines, and PMS. Dab onto wrists and temples, breathe in, and close your eyes.

Add carrier oil to small spouted measuring cup. With separate eyedroppers, add essential oils to carrier oil and combine with spoon. With funnel, pour slowly into roll-on bottles. Press on roll-on lid and screw on cap.

Use as needed. If stored out of direct sunlight, will keep for up to 2 years.

YIELD: ½ OUNCE

INGREDIENTS

1 tablespoon carrier oil of choice

8 drops peppermint essential oil

7 drops eucalyptus essential oil

5 drops clary sage essential oil

3 drops rosemary essential oil

Optional: 5 drops lavender essential oil*

* Use if you or your friends love lavender; some people don't.

Sweet Rest Calming Blend

YIELD: ½ OUNCE

INGREDIENTS

1 tablespoon carrier oil of choice

7 drops sweet orange essential oil

5 drops frankincense essential oil

5 drops rose geranium
essential oil

4 drops chamomile essential oil

When you are winding down for bed or need to calm your nerves, this calming blend will soothe your senses and help you rest. Dab onto wrists and temples, breathe in, and close your eyes.

———————————————

Add carrier oil to small spouted measuring cup. With separate eyedroppers, add essential oils to carrier oil and combine with spoon. With funnel, pour slowly into roll-on bottles. Press on roll-on lid and screw on cap.

Use as needed. If stored out of direct sunlight, will keep for up to 2 years.

Forest Sprite Grounding Blend

YIELD: ½ OUNCE

INGREDIENTS

1 tablespoon carrier oil of choice

4 drops fir balsam essential oil

4 drops vetiver essential oil

3 drops juniper berry essential oil

3 drops clary sage essential oil

This blend is a grounding, experiential scent that smells earthy and green. Perfect when you need focus or if you want to smell woodsy. Dab onto wrists and temples, sniff, and focus.

———————————————

Add carrier oil to small spouted measuring cup. With separate eyedroppers, add essential oils to carrier oil and combine with spoon. With funnel, pour slowly into roll-on bottles. Press on roll-on lid and screw on cap.

Use as needed. If stored out of direct sunlight, will keep for up to 2 years.

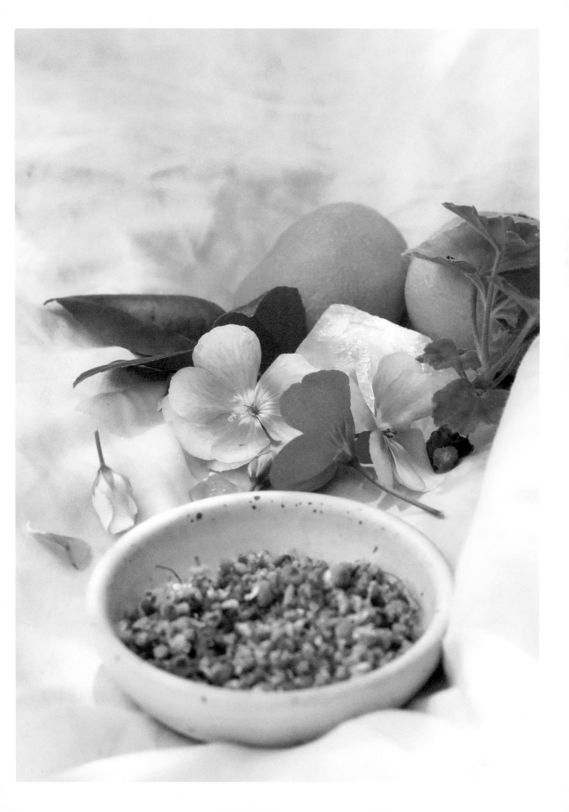

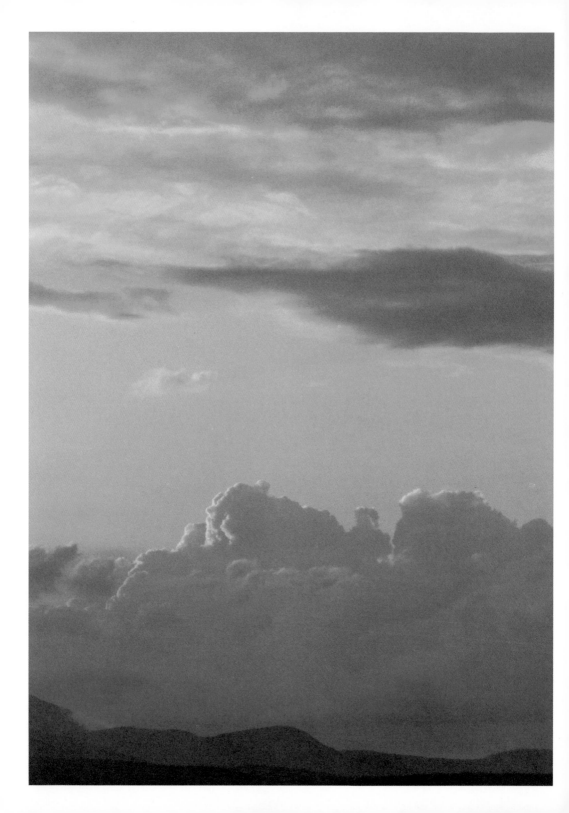

Deep Breath Calming Spray

I love this spray to take things down a notch any time of day. You can mist it on your face and body for calming, followed by some deep breaths. It is also great to prepare children for rest time. Spray it on pillows or in the air before bedtime for you and your whole family.

———————————————

Combine all ingredients in measuring cup; stir with spoon. Pour into 4-ounce glass bottle and screw on sprayer.

Shake well before use and spray as desired. If stored out of direct sunlight, will keep for up to 6 months. Adding alcohol will keep the spray fresh for up to a year.

YIELD: 4 OUNCES

INGREDIENTS

4 ounces distilled water

30 drops sweet orange essential oil

20 drops chamomile essential oil

15 drops lavender essential oil

Optional: 1 teaspoon high-proof alcohol

Emerald Green Woods Room Spray

A walk in the woods in a bottle. Green, fresh, and mind clearing, it works well as a linen or sweater spray to refresh fabrics or create a forest cloak.

———————————————

Combine all ingredients in measuring cup; stir with spoon. Pour into 4-ounce glass bottle and screw on sprayer.

Shake well before use and spray as desired. If stored out of direct sunlight, will keep for up to 6 months. Adding alcohol will keep the spray fresh for up to a year.

YIELD: 4 OUNCES

INGREDIENTS

4 ounces distilled water

30 drops fir needle essential oil

20 drops juniper berry essential oil

10 drops vetiver essential oil

Optional: 1 teaspoon high-proof alcohol

Good Vibrations Clearing Spray

YIELD: 4 OUNCES

INGREDIENTS

4 ounces distilled water

20 drops lime essential oil

15 drops eucalyptus essential oil

10 drops white sage essential oil

Optional: 1 teaspoon
high-proof alcohol

This spray is designed to help you clear energy and set intentions. Since it is formulated as an alternative to smudging, you can spray it liberally on yourself, in your space, and wherever you feel needs some cleansing. I personally like the ritual of spraying it around myself at the beginning of a new day.

————————————

Combine all ingredients in measuring cup; stir with spoon. Pour into 4-ounce glass bottle and screw on sprayer.

Shake well before use and spray as desired. If stored out of direct sunlight, will keep for up to 6 months. Adding alcohol will keep the spray fresh for up to a year.

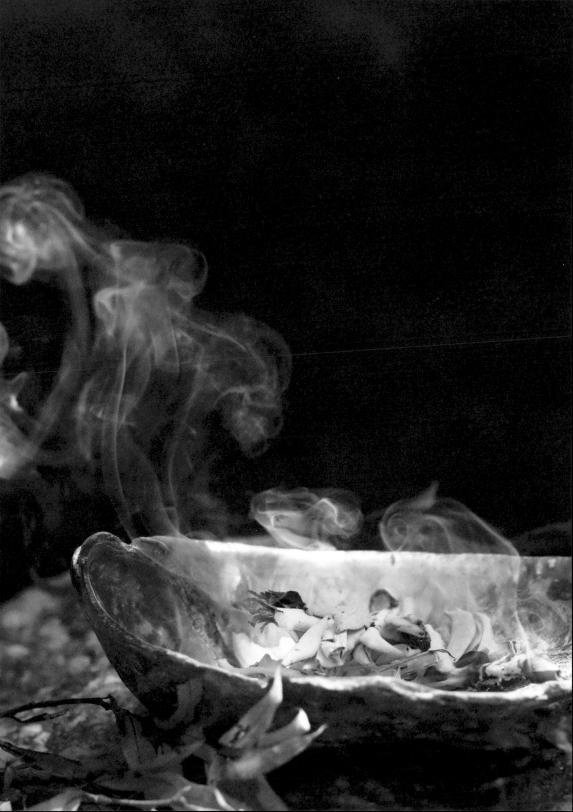

CHAPTER THREE

Pursuing Wild Beauty

"When we accept our own wild beauty, it is put into perspective. . . .
Does a wolf know how beautiful she is when she leaps? Does a feline
know what beautiful shapes she makes when she sits? Is a bird awed by
the sound it hears when it snaps open its wings? Learning from them, we
just act in our own true way and do not draw back from or hide our
natural beauty. Like the creatures, we just are, and it is right." [11]

Clarissa Pinkola Estés, *Women Who Run with the Wolves*

As you can probably sense about me so far, I like to know what I am putting on and into my body. Like Michael Pollan's seminal mantra about food, "Eat food, not too much, mostly plants," I would echo this for beauty—"Use products, not very much, mostly from plants." I relish in the beauty of plant- and mineral-based ingredients. Their names read like a poem: aloe, sea kelp, witch hazel, rose, blue chamomile. On the other hand, there is nothing sexy about Cetaphil. It is made of water, cetyl alcohol, propylene glycol, sodium lauryl sulfate, stearyl alcohol, methylparaben, propylparaben, and butylparaben. Shouldn't you be excited about and relish in the ingredients that are nourishing your skin?

As a very visual person, I like to read ingredient lists and visualize the plants those ingredients come from. Isn't it more beautiful to imagine geranium, rose, or coconut than petrochemicals made from petroleum, natural gas, or coal? It might just be me, but does anything seem less appetizing for your skin than petroleum jelly? The raw material for petroleum jelly was discovered in America in 1859. It came from—you guessed it—petroleum. The story of how it was discovered is equally unappealing. Workers on the country's first oil rigs disliked the black paraffin-like substance forming on their equipment until they discovered it seemed to have healing properties. This by-product of petroleum production was taken into a laboratory, refined, and, voilà, the iconic Vaseline petroleum jelly was born. Slathered all over babies' bottoms, people's bodies, and hair is a product made from crude oil.

Shea butter is actually a natural substitute for petroleum jelly, which is an occlusive moisturizer, meaning it prevents water loss in skin by creating a barrier and locking in moisture. Shea butter has this same quality naturally and is a wonderful emollient, both softening and nourishing the skin. Instead of petroleum, shea butter comes from the nuts of the *Vitellaria paradoxa* tree and has been used by the people of East and West Africa on skin, hair, and nails for centuries. It contains anti-inflammatory and antioxidant properties and literally melts on skin, unlike the sticky, gooey petroleum jelly. Our body is not a car. It deserves to be treated with care. That's why I choose plant oils over crude oil.

People often think that switching from conventional products both for self-care and the home is unattainably expensive. I beg to differ. If we become more conscious as consumers and decrease the amount we consume, we will not only save money but will also help our planet. We supersize our food, supersize our products, and consume with abandon. Less is more. If we buy quality products and use them with care, they are well worth the price. We can also choose to make them ourselves with very simple, healthful ingredients.

The way we treat ourselves is a much bigger part of our beauty than what we put on our skin. Wild beauty is the powerful acceptance to be fully ourselves. Silver hair is beautiful just as silver foxes are beautiful. Lines give character just like the veins of crystal in a rock. You are a natural wonder.

I believe in skin, hair, and body care that nourishes and enhances our beauty naturally. It should be a pleasure to use. Just as you would not swallow something that tastes bad, please never use anything on your body that doesn't smell or feel good to you. In this chapter, we are going to dive into ingredient lists; demystify products such as toner and face oil; investigate plant-based ingredients; and highlight some of the nasty ones I think you should avoid.

Demystifying Ingredient Lists

Ingredient lists are quantitative: they are listed in order from the highest-percentage ingredient to the lowest one. We often focus on the first ingredients on the list, but often we fail to pay sufficient attention to the ingredients lower on the list. If we see aloe vera listed at the top, we might grab the bottle and not see "fragrance" lurking below. Of course, this means it is a lesser ingredient in the formula, but it is still a potent and potentially hazardous ingredient.

When I started my company, I had no idea about the regulations for listing ingredients. I was always baffled why ingredient lists would include the Latin name of the ingredient, thus making it more obscure for the consumer. As I got further along with the business, I came to understand that the botanical or International Nomenclature of Cosmetic Ingredients (INCI) name is a standardized way to communicate across language barriers the exact ingredients that are in a product. While the common name, shea butter, might be more easily recognizable and sound more appealing than *Butyrospermum parkii*, the Latin or scientific name is the rule that transcends culture.

If you ever are mystified by an ingredient's INCI name, it is a quick search away on the internet or the Environmental Working Group Skin Deep app or website (www.ewg.org/skindeep).

NOTHING LASTS FOREVER

There is a strange belief that products should last forever, or at least for years. We buy perishable fresh food but somehow expect ingredients in our beauty products to be invincible. Less is more doesn't apply only to how busy we make our lives but also to how much we consume. We live in a culture of more is more is more. Just like the food we consume, products shouldn't last forever. Synthetic chemical preservatives are often added to beauty products to make them last longer. For ultimate freshness, I always recommend using a product within six months if you can. Look for products that have natural preservatives, like vitamin E, essential oils (including rosemary, thyme, and eucalyptus), radish root ferment filtrate, or food-grade preservatives such as sea salt, citric acid, or potassium sorbate.

A NOTE ON TOWELS & DRY BRUSHING

All towels are not the same. Choose organic cotton or gently exfoliating organic fiber washcloths to wash your face. Look for soft organic towels or cloths for your body and hair.

Instead of those creepy-colored, jellyfish-looking plastic sponges, opt for a sustainably harvested, natural sea wool sponge. Sea wool sponges are biodegradable and the perfect way to naturally cleanse and exfoliate skin.

Dry brushing is also a powerful practice for smoother skin and lymphatic massage. It helps exfoliate and rejuvenate our skin. Dry brushing has many additional benefits, including helping boost your immune system, improve circulation, and aid digestion. Use light pressure and brush your dry body in small strokes or a circular motion always headed toward your heart. Use a cactus-bristle brush, and be careful with your body, you should always plan to shower or bathe after dry brushing to remove dead skin.

NAMES TELL A STORY

The fascinating thing about Latin names for species, be they animal, mineral, or plant, is that they tell a story. The story could be the person who discovered it, the place it was found, or a characteristic of the species.

Here are a few of my favorite plant names that are among the essential oils I discuss in this book.

Chamomile (*Chamaemelum nobile*)
Chamaemelum: from *chamae*, which means low to the ground, and *mel* for honey, evocative of the smell.
Nobile: noble

Geranium (*Pelargonium graveolens*)
Pelargonium: from *pelargos*, which means "stork," and *gonium*, referring to the shape of a stork's bill.
Graveolens: heavily scented

Lavender (*Lavandula angustifolia*)
Lavandula: from the verb *lavare*, "to wash." Historically, the scent was used to freshen laundry.
Angustifolia: narrow-leaved

Rosemary (*Rosmarinus officinalis*)
Rosmarinus: rose of the sea
Officinalis: used officially in medicine

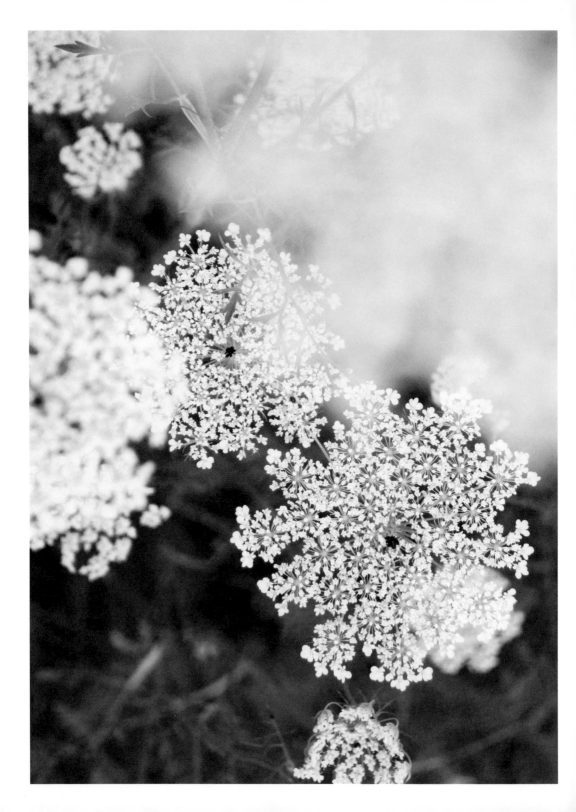

If you want to avoid synthetic chemicals in beauty products, the most important thing you can do is learn to read ingredient lists. Here, I will outline some of my favorite ingredients to look for and some of the ones I think it would be best to avoid.

Ingredients I Love

Activated charcoal or activated carbon is used both externally and internally to detoxify skin and body. It has been heated to increase absorptive properties. Activated charcoal has long been used at hospitals or at home as an antidote for poisoning and overdoses. It attaches to toxins and absorbs them before they enter the bloodstream. For skin, charcoal has the ability to draw out dirt, impurities, pollution, and chemicals so you can wash them away. It is great for all skin types but particularly oily skin. It is perfect in a cleanser or face mask and is also used in toothpaste to whiten teeth.

Aloe vera (*Aloe barbadensis*) is the green spined succulent that thrives in tropical landscapes but can happily live in your home as well. Popularly known as a sunburn remedy, aloe vera is so much more. It was regarded by ancient Egyptians as the plant of immortality for its healing properties. Aloe vera is full of antioxidants, vitamins, minerals, enzymes, amino acids, and salicylic acid. It is used both internally and externally to soothe and cool. For skin and body, aloe vera is effective at moisturizing, relieving rashes and skin irritations, and healing burns, wounds, and dry skin. For hair, aloe hydrates, adds subtle holding power, and has been used as a remedy for hair loss. Aloe vera is the ultimate refresher; it is a great addition to personal care products to add natural hydration and moisture.

To create aloe vera gel, remove the outer leaf and cold press or blend the slimy inner substance into a smooth gel. If you buy aloe vera gel, make sure the only preservatives it contains are foodgrade ones such as citric acid and potassium sorbate.

Apple cider vinegar is not only a delight in salad dressing, it is an incredible ingredient for skin and hair care. It is anti-inflammatory and astringent, and it helps balance the pH of your skin. The smell can be a bit challenging for some, but you can tone it down with essential oils and hydrosols.

Castile soap is a natural cleanser made by saponifying, or turning into soap, plant oils such as olive oil, coconut, sunflower, and jojoba, with the addition of potassium hydroxide. Gentle and effective, castile soap is great for washing face, body, and hair and can be used in household cleaners.

Clay has played an integral role in history. It has been used since ancient times for building homes and creating eating vessels, as well as for internal and external use. For our skin, clay is an important detox tool. With both cleansing and exfoliating properties, it draws toxins and impurities out of the skin. Mixed into a paste with water or hydrosol, it is the perfect face mask or mud bath.

The most popular clays in beauty and personal care products are kaolin, bentonite, French green clay, rhassoul clay, or pink clay.

Fruit enzymes are nature's answer to a chemical peel. The natural enzymes found in fruits such as apple, blueberry, grapes, kiwi, lemon, lime, pineapple, papaya, and pumpkin help naturally exfoliate and slough off dead skin cells, resulting in softer and smoother skin.

Honey not only tastes delicious, but it is perhaps the oldest beauty ingredient. Throughout time, it has been used for its internal and external healing abilities. It is naturally emollient, humectant, antibacterial, and full of antioxidants. Use it straight out of the honeypot to cleanse skin, and add it to masks and moisturizers. It is also great for acne prevention and treatment as well as for dry skin as it both soothes and seals in moisture. Always make sure the honey you buy is raw, unpasteurized, and local when possible.

Manuka honey is a special type of honey from New Zealand made by bees that pollinate the manuka bush. It has a higher antibacterial quality than ordinary honey and is a delight to eat or use for skin conditions and wound healing.

Maple syrup is a great vegan alternative to honey in recipes. This sweet super-power ingredient has a high antioxidant content similar to that of raw honey.

Sea salt is a wonderful natural exfoliant that helps slough off dead skin cells. It adds volume and texture to hair in a sea salt spray. Sea salt contains potassium, which helps prevent and ease muscle pain, cramps, and stress. Dissolved into a bath, it is an ideal way to unwind and the perfect remedy for a tired, sore body. Think of it as the ocean in your bath; add a little seaweed and voilà! Sea salt is also a natural preservative.

Seaweed brings us back to the primacy of the ocean. It is an incredibly nutritious food, high in iodine, vitamins, and minerals. It is also incredibly beneficial to our skin. Some common seaweeds that are wonderful both as food and in beauty products are kelp (*Macrocystis pyrifera*), bladderwrack (*Fucus vesiculosus*), and Irish moss (*Chondrus crispus*).

Witch hazel (*Hamamelis virginiana*) is a natural astringent distilled from the leaves and bark of the witch hazel tree. It grows throughout the eastern United States and has fragrant yellow flowers that bloom in the fall. It has long been used for its medicinal properties to disinfect and treat skin irritations and is an important part of a natural first-aid kit. Witch hazel is great straight out of the bottle as a toner for all skin types. Most witch hazel you purchase has alcohol added to it for stability. If you want a purer product, purchase witch hazel hydrosol or distillate.

Yogurt contains natural lactic acid that helps regenerate skin and balance skin pH. It also feels incredibly soothing for skin. It is high in antioxidants, helps fight free radicals, and is antibacterial, making it perfect for all skin types. Try washing your skin with yogurt or using a yogurt mask. Both soy and coconut yogurt contain lactic acid and are great vegan alternatives.

CARRIER OILS

Argan (*Argania spinosa*) is produced from the kernels of the nuts from the argan tree native to Morocco. This incredibly precious oil is made through a laborious process that involves removing the nuts from the fruit of the tree by hand, cracking them, and removing the kernels from the nut (nuts typically contain one to three kernels). Then the kernels are cold-pressed into oil. Argan oil is often referred to as liquid gold because of its ability to treat a variety of skin and hair conditions. As with many valuable minerals, extraction is a lengthy process.

My mother grew up in Morocco, so I have long been steeped in the culinary and cosmetic delights of argan oil. It provides lightweight moisture, is easily absorbed by skin and hair, and is high in vitamin E and fatty acids. It is a great base or addition to a face or hair oil.

Coconut oil (*Cocos nucifera*) is a delicious treat to taste, smell, and feel. Made from pressing raw coconut meat, the oil, which smells like fresh coconut, is a sumptuous moisturizer for skin and hair. Solid at room temperature, coconut oil can be scooped right from the container onto your skin. Coconut oil has the ability to strengthen skin tissues, improving elasticity. It is high in antioxidants and vitamin E, as well as fatty acids, including lauric acid, a natural microbial. It is often used in both solid and liquid soaps for its ability to produce a lovely lather. I love it blended with cocoa butter to create a natural "Mounds bar" for your skin. Make sure you buy raw, virgin, and unrefined coconut oil for the best experience.

Sunflower seed oil (*Helianthus annuus*) is an inexpensive but great option for face, body, and hair oils. It is high in oleic acid, a fatty acid found in the human body, which makes it ideal for nourishing dry skin. It is also high in antioxidant-rich vitamin E.

Jojoba oil (*Simmondsia chinensis*) is the closest oil to our own sebum. It is technically not an oil but rather a wax ester. Waxes help seal in moisture, so this makes jojoba a perfect choice for adding moisture and locking it in at the same time. A great base for a face, body, or hair oil or for oil-based perfume.

Rosehip seed oil (*Rosa canina*) oil is pressed from the tiny seeds inside rosehips of the *Rosa canina* or "dog rose." A deeply nourishing oil, it is easily absorbed by the skin and ranges in color from amber to rich orange-red. It is high in vitamins A, C, and E as well as three essential fatty acids and is a luxurious addition to face oil, especially for dry, mature skin.

Sea buckthorn oil (*Hippophae rhamnoides*) is made from the sour orange berries of a shrub native to Asia and Europe. This precious oil, known for its rejuvenative properties, is great for all skin types. It is a highly concentrated, powerful oil that can be added in small doses to skin-care preparations. The orange-red color comes from a high concentration of beta-carotene. It is also high in vitamins A, C, E, and K, as well as omega-3 fatty acids. I love adding a few drops to face oils, hair oil, scalp treatments, spot serums, or eye serums. It can also be taken internally to help with dry skin.

BUTTERS

Cocoa butter (*Theobroma cacao*) is as good as it sounds, tastes, and smells. This tasty natural fat, which adds smoothness and mouth-melting appeal to a piece of chocolate, also has the same benefits for your skin. The cacao bean has been used for centuries in Central and South America and the Caribbean not only for making chocolate but in skin-care preparations. Cocoa butter is high in essential fatty acids and antioxidants and is a natural emollient, helping to seal in moisture. It is ideal for all skin types, including sensitive or dry skin and cracked lips; plus it helps prevent and heal stretch marks. It smells like dark chocolate and is edible. It is hard and brittle at room temperature. I like to melt it and whip with shea butter and coconut oil for a sumptuous treat for skin. Make sure you buy virgin, unrefined cocoa butter that hasn't been deodorized. I know! Why on Earth would anyone want to deodorize it?

Shea butter (*Butyrospermum parkii*) is made from the nuts of the shea (karite) tree in Africa. It is high in vitamins A, E, and F; provides collagen; and is a natural emollient. It has a natural SPF of 6. A miracle treatment for dry skin, lips, body, and scalp, shea butter helps with skin elasticity. Virgin, unrefined shea butter has a mild nutty smell and is soft and pliable at room temperature.

WAXES

Beeswax (*Cera alba*) is a natural wax produced by honeybees. Female worker bees create beeswax through the consumption of honey that they turn into wax through special wax-producing glands. The wax they create is composed of esters of fatty acids and various long-chain alcohols. Always look for golden beeswax if you are using it in products; white beeswax has been bleached.

Candelilla wax (*Euphorbia cerifera*) is a plant-based wax made from the Mexican candelilla plant. It is a great vegan alternative to beeswax. It is a little bit harder than beeswax and imparts a beautiful gloss to products.

Ingredients to Avoid

The European Union has banned 1,300 ingredients in personal care products while the United States has banned a paltry 30. The US Food and Drug Administration does not actively regulate the personal care or cosmetics industries, so unfortunately consumers have to take matters into their own hands. Even if you do your due diligence, companies do not have to disclose ingredients that are classified as trade secrets. The need for transparency is dire. My two cents is to shop only with companies that disclose their ingredients and whose values you believe in.

This is in no way a comprehensive list of all the toxic ingredients that can be found in products, but some of the top dirty ingredients you should look out for.

Butane is also known as lighter fluid. This highly flammable, liquefiable gas made from petroleum is found in many skin, body, and hair products and even in food! It is used in antiperspirants, deodorants, hair spray, perfume, shaving cream, tanning products, and aerosol products such as some dry shampoos. It is potentially carcinogenic, dangerous to inhale, and could cause your hair to catch fire.

Coal tar and its derivatives are obtained through the distillation of coal. This thick substance is used to color cosmetics and hair dyes and also ends up in over-the-counter dandruff, psoriasis. and eczema products. This is strange, since coal tar is linked to allergic skin reactions, including rashes and hives. It also causes organ-system toxicity and cancer in animals and is an environmental toxin.

Diazolidinyl urea is an antimicrobial preservative that releases formaldehyde. It is a common but toxic ingredient in personal-care items.

Formaldehyde is the same substance that is used to preserve dead animals, and it is found in products ranging from nail polish to soap to eye drops. It is an odorless gas used as a hardening agent in nail polish, a preservative, as well as a disinfectant. It causes allergic reactions, skin sensitivity, and irritation and is carcinogenic. Many other ingredients such as diazolidinyl urea and quaternium-15 release formaldehyde.

Hydroquinone is an antioxidant that is used in skin bleach, hair color, and fragrances. It can cause skin depigmentation, allergic reactions, and organ system toxicity.

Parabens are the most common preservatives used in the United States. Methylparaben and propylparaben appear in up to 90 percent of products, including shampoo, conditioner, body washes, lotions, and sunscreens. Parabens have estrogen-like properties and have been linked to breast cancer.

Petrochemicals (PC) are found in almost all conventional beauty products in one way or another. You want to avoid petroleum in your products for countless reasons. Here is a list of some of the most common petrochemicals you can find in beauty products:

BENZENE

BUTYL WORDS
(E.G., BUTYLENE GLYCOL)

DIETHANOLAMINE (DEA)

-ETH WORDS (E.G., LAURETH)

ETHANOLAMINE (MEA)

METHYL WORDS
(E.G., METHYLPARABEN)

MINERAL OIL

PARAFFIN WAX

POLYETHYLENE GLYCOL (PEG)

PETROLEUM JELLY

PHENOXYETHANOL

PROPYL WORDS
(E.G., PROPYLENE GLYCOL)

TOLUENE

Phthlates are used to give flexibility to plastic and serve the same function in personal care items and cosmetics. They also help extend the scent of perfume. The most common phthalates found in products are diethyl phthalate (DEP), dimethyl phthalate (DMP), and dibutyl phthalate (DBP).

Propylene glycol is used as antifreeze and engine coolant and is also one of the most widely used ingredients in personal care products. You can find it in makeup, sunscreen, baby products, deodorants, aftershave, creams, and mouthwash. It is a preservative, humectant, and solvent. It has been linked to eye, skin, and lung irritation as well as organ system toxicity.

Retinyl palmitate is made of the ester of vitamin A and palmitic acid. It is widely used for antioxidant properties in skin care, hair care, body care, and nail and sunscreen products. A major issue is that studies show that retinyl palmitate can spur excess skin growth (hyperplasia) as well as form free radicals when exposed to sunlight.

Synthetic surfactants are used to reduce the surface tension of water in a formula to allow it to slip, spread, foam, or emulsify. Surfactants show up in products such as body wash, shaving cream, face and body lotion, shampoo, conditioner, and toothpaste. Castile soap is an example of a natural surfactant, but most surfactants are synthetic and derived from sources such as petroleum. Other naturally derived gentle surfactant alternatives are coconut-derived coco glucoside, decyl glucoside, and decyl polyglucoside.

The following synthetic surfactants are used in personal care products. They are allergens and skin irritants that are potential endocrine disrupters and carcinogens, and they have been linked to liver organ toxicity:

AMMONIUM LAURETH SULFATE (ALES)

AMMONIUM LAURYL SULFATE (ALS)

DISODIUM DIOCTYL SULFOSUCCINATE

DISODIUM LAURETH SULFOSUCCINATE

DISODIUM OLEAMIDE SULFOSUCCINATE

DIETHANOLAMINE (DEA)

LAURYL OR COCOYL SARCOSINE

MONOETHANOLAMINE (MEA)

POLYETHYLENE GLYCOL (PEG)

POLYPROPYLENE GLYCOL (PPG)

POTASSIUM COCOYL HYDROLYZED COLLAGEN

QUATERNIUM-7, -15, -31, -60

SODIUM COCOYL SARCOSINATE

SODIUM LAURETH SULFATE (SLES)

SODIUM LAUROYL SARCOSINATE

SODIUM LAURYL SULFATE (SLS)

SODIUM METHYL COCOYL TAURATE

TRIETHANOLAMINE (TEA)

Talc is the finely ground mineral magnesium silicate. It is a common ingredient in baby powders, body powders, face powders, foot powders, eye shadow, and dry shampoo. Talc is dangerous if inhaled, because it has similar properties to asbestos. Talcum powder has been linked to ovarian cancer in women who have used it as a body powder, because it can enter the reproductive areas. Natural and safe alternatives include cornstarch and arrowroot powder.

Toluene is a petrochemical ingredient used in gasoline. It is also found in nail products and hair dyes. It has been linked to skin and lung irritation, reproductive system toxicity, and organ system toxicity.

Triclosan and **triclocarban** were common ingredients in antibacterial soaps until they were recently banned by the FDA.

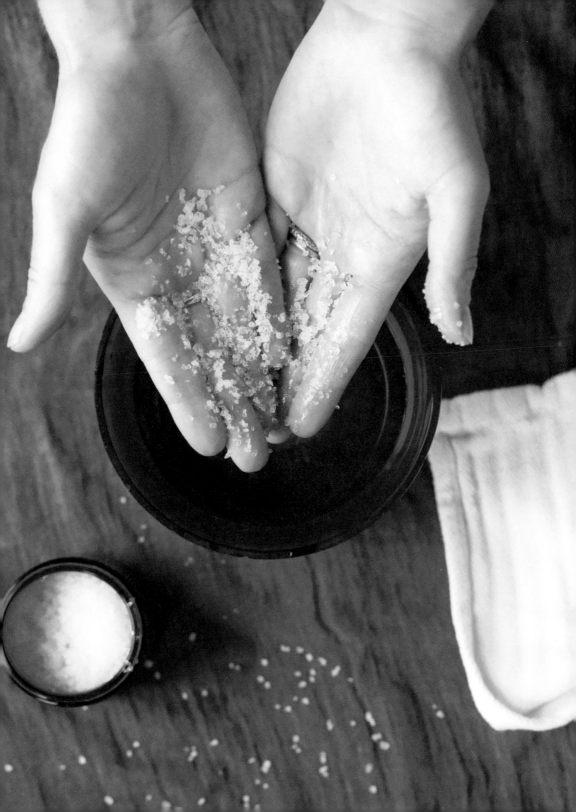

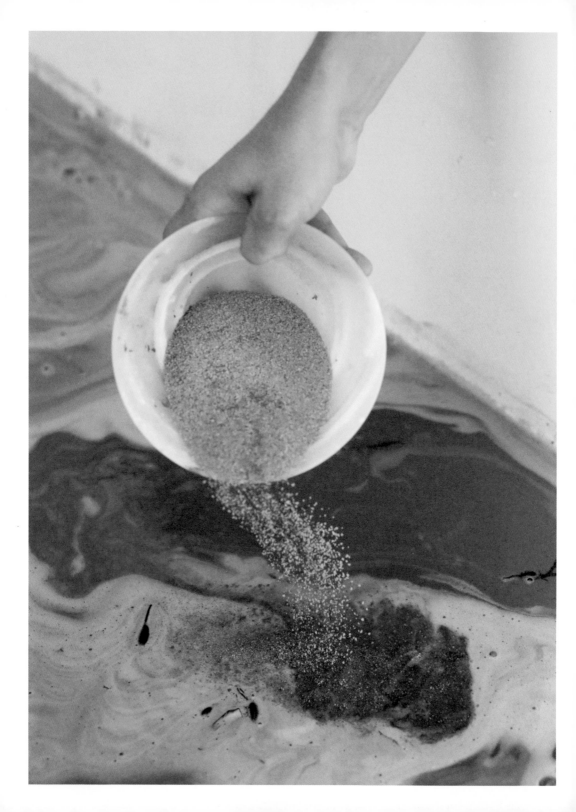

Emerald Sea Detox Bath

This dreamy green bath will envelop your senses and balance your body. Nourishing sea kelp stimulates blood flow and draws impurities out of skin. Antioxidant-rich spirulina fights free radicals, retains moisture, and creates a beautiful jade-green hue over the bath. Epsom salt relieves tired muscles and eliminates toxins, while mineral-rich sea salt balances skin moisture and improves circulation.

Mix all ingredients together in bowl and stir well. Spoon into jar and close with lid.

Use ¼ to ½ cup per bath or as desired. Will keep fresh for up to a year.

YIELD: 16 OUNCES

INGREDIENTS

1 cup sea salt

1 cup Epsom salt

2 tablespoons green clay or bentonite clay

¼ cup kelp powder

¼ cup spirulina powder

20 drops eucalyptus or lemongrass essential oil

ADDITIONAL EQUIPMENT

16-ounce jar with lid

Aquamarine Bubble Bath

This brings back memories of childhood and getting treated to a big foamy bath in my parents' tub. There are few ingredients, but they are more than a sum of their parts. If you have jets in your tub, use them for extra foam.

Mix all ingredients together in measuring cup and pour into bottle with lid.

Use 2 ounces or as desired in bath. Will keep for up to a year.

YIELD: 8 OUNCES

INGREDIENTS

1 cup castile soap

10 drops fir balsam essential oil

10 drops neroli essential oil

Optional: 1 teaspoon spirulina*

* Add this directly to the bath water for an aquamarine hue.

ADDITIONAL EQUIPMENT

8-ounce glass bottle with lid

Hydrating Body Wash

YIELD: 8 OUNCES

INGREDIENTS

2 tablespoons shea butter

½ cup aloe vera

1 teaspoon vitamin E

Scent options:

20 drops rose geranium
essential oil

10 drops vetiver essential oil

10 drops eucalyptus essential oil

15 drops fir balsam essential oil

½ cup castile soap

ADDITIONAL EQUIPMENT

8-ounce glass bottle with lid

A simple but rich recipe that uses castile soap as a base and mixes it with nourishing shea butter and soothing aloe vera. This soap is a delight to the skin and the senses and will easily become part of your bathing ritual. This makes a concentrated, very sudsy soap that is great when used with a sea sponge. You can also dilute with more aloe or water as desired.

Heat 2 inches of water in small pot over medium heat. Once it boils, turn down to simmer.

Add shea butter to heatproof cup or bowl and put in pot. Once shea butter melts, remove from heat and let cool.

Once cool, add aloe vera, vitamin E, and essential oils and blend on low speed with immersion blender for 30 seconds. Add castile soap and stir in with spoon. Pour mixture into bottle with lid.

Use in bath or shower. If stored out of direct sunlight, will keep for up to 6 months.

No-More-Scales Body Oil

This deeply nourishing body oil is great year-round for keeping your body soft, nourished, and glowing. This powerful mix of carrier oils and essential oils will make your skin sing. Use right after shower on damp skin for best absorption. Can also be used as shaving oil.

———————————

Mix all ingredients together in small mixing bowl and stir well with spoon. Pour into bottle with lid.

Use generously on damp skin after shower or as desired. If stored out of direct sunlight, will keep for up to a year.

YIELD: 8 OUNCES

INGREDIENTS

¾ cup sunflower oil

¼ cup jojoba oil

½ teaspoon sea buckthorn oil

For a fresh floral scent:

15 drops lavender essential oil

10 drops lemongrass essential oil

For a green, springy scent:

25 drops rose geranium essential oil

20 drops juniper berry essential oil

ADDITIONAL EQUIPMENT

8-ounce glass bottle with pump or lid

Dream-Cream Deodorant

YIELD: 4 OUNCES

INGREDIENTS

¼ cup coconut oil

2 tablespoons shea butter

¼ cup arrowroot powder
or cornstarch

¼ cup baking soda (or use
magnesium hydroxide if you
are baking-soda sensitive)

About 25 drops essential oil
blend of your choice*

Optional: 1 tablespoon
beeswax or vegan wax**

* Scent options:

7 drops sage and
20 drops fir balsam

15 drops geranium and
10 drops lemon

** Otherwise, deodorant
will be soft in texture.

ADDITIONAL EQUIPMENT

4-ounce glass jar, or two 2-ounce
glass jars, with lid(s)

I always say deodorant is the first product you should select for a clean swap. Conventional deodorants and antiperspirants contain aluminum and synthetic fragrance. Our armpits are a very absorptive area of our bodies because of the number of sweat glands. Antiperspirants inhibit our body's natural ability to sweat, which prevents us from releasing toxins. Conventional deodorants are really the pits. This natural cream deodorant made with a few simple ingredients fights bacteria, moisture, and odor and soothes armpits.

Heat 3 inches of water in small pot over medium heat. Once it boils, turn down to simmer.

Add coconut oil, shea butter, and wax (if using) to measuring cup and put in pot. Once coconut oil, shea butter, and wax melt, remove from heat and let cool until warm but not hot to the touch. Add arrowroot powder and baking soda into mixture; stir well. Add essential oils and stir again. Pour into jar(s) and let solidify. (If you choose not to use wax, you might need to pop your deodorant into the fridge periodically if it melts.)

If stored out of direct sunlight, will keep for up to a year.

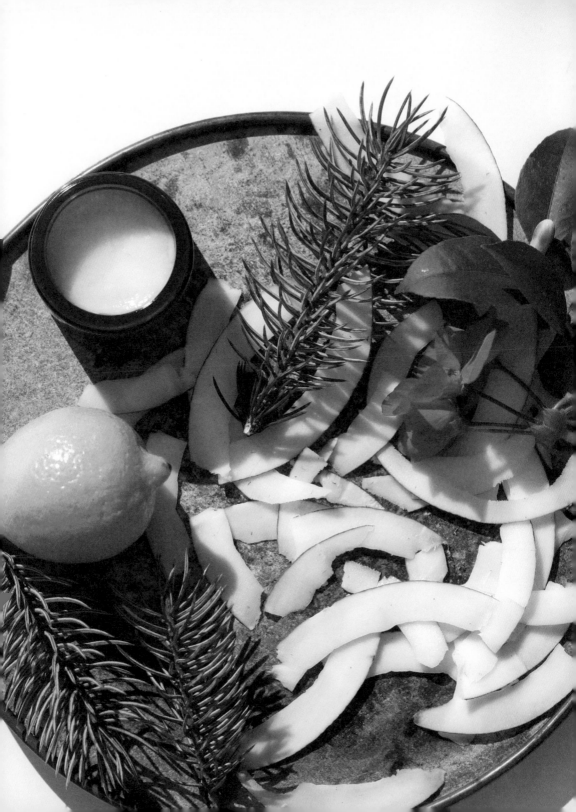

Cocoa-Nut Body Butter

YIELD: 8 OUNCES

INGREDIENTS

¼ cup shea butter

¼ cup cocoa butter

½ cup coconut oil

Optional: ½ teaspoon vitamin E

ADDITIONAL EQUIPMENT

Stand mixer or blender
with whisk attachment

Spatula

8-ounce glass jar or two
4-ounce glass jars, with lid(s)

This stuff is the best. Creamy, dreamy, and a delight to the senses because it smells like chocolate and coconut. This is a simple but decadent recipe that will keep your skin soft all year long. Safe to use on the whole family, even babies.

———————————

Heat 3 inches of water in pot over medium heat. Once it boils, turn down to simmer.

Add shea butter, cocoa butter, coconut oil, and vitamin E (if using) to measuring cup and put in pot. Stir occasionally with spoon until fully melted. Remove from heat. When glass is lukewarm to touch, put mixture in refrigerator with small plate on top (to protect mixture). Leave for 1 or 2 hours until cool.

Prepare stand mixer or use blender with whisk attachment. Scoop mixture out of measuring cup and into mixing bowl. Whisk at medium speed for 10 minutes. When cream sticks to sides, push down with spatula to reintegrate. When mixture is fluffy, remove bowl from mixer and scrape into jar. Seal with lid.

Use as desired with clean, dry fingers. (If cream gets soft, pop into refrigerator for an hour.) If stored out of direct sunlight, will keep for up to a year.

Fly & Tick Spray

Where we live, the ticks are terrible from spring through fall, and the rose geranium and peppermint essential oils in this spray keep them away. Lemon eucalyptus essential oil is a highly effective way to ward off mosquitoes and flies, as are lemongrass and cedarwood essential oils. Can be sprayed on children and dogs.

Mix all ingredients together in measuring cup. Pour mixture into bottle with fine-mist sprayer.

Shake well before use. Spray liberally on your skin, clothes, and hair before going outside. If stored out of direct sunlight, will keep for up to a year.

YIELD: 4 OUNCES

INGREDIENTS

½ cup witch hazel

15 drops lemon eucalyptus essential oil

15 drops rose geranium essential oil

10 drops lemongrass essential oil

10 drops peppermint essential oil

5 drops cedarwood essential oil

ADDITIONAL EQUIPMENT

4-ounce bottle with fine-mist sprayer

Sea Salt & Sunshine Body Scrub

YIELD: 8 OUNCES

INGREDIENTS

1 cup fine sea salt, or mix of fine and medium grain

¼ cup coconut oil, or more as desired

½ teaspoon vitamin E

20 drops sweet orange essential oil

10 drops lemongrass essential oil

Optional: 1 tablespoon shea butter

ADDITIONAL EQUIPMENT

8-ounce glass jar with lid

A good salt scrub is a necessity in my opinion. Mineral-rich sea salt helps exfoliate skin, slough off dead skin cells, helps with cell regeneration, reduces inflammation, and improves circulation. Dry, flaky skin becomes soft and glowing. Coconut oil adds moisture and is delightful combined with sweet orange essential oil. This is great to use before shaving for a much smoother shave. I also love this for exfoliating lips when they are dry and chapped.

Mix ingredients together in bowl with spoon. (If coconut oil is hard, you can melt quickly and add to mixture once cool. If you want to add shea butter for even more nourishment, do the same thing.) Once mixed, with spoon, scoop scrub into jar with lid.

Use once or twice weekly or as desired; by rubbing salt with dry, clean fingers in circular motion all over body and feet. Rinse well. If stored out of direct sunlight, will keep for up to a year (if water is kept out of jar).

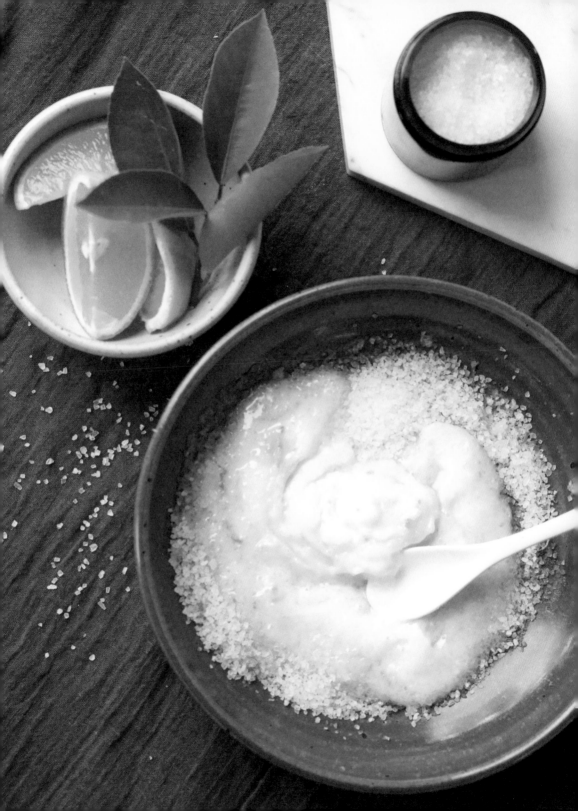

CHAPTER FOUR

Skin

"There's no need to imagine that you're a wondrous beauty, because that's what you are."[12]

Tove Jansson, *Moominsummer Madness*

O ur skin is not only our largest organ but it is also the most visible one. Like any other organ in our bodies, our skin is affected by how we treat it. When our faces are dry and inflamed or we break out, we don't want to show this to the world. Our reaction is usually to hide under heavy makeup, but this can make things worse. The key is to try to treat the problem holistically. Chances are that it is a combination of both internal and external factors.

Oil Essentials

There is a myth that oil is bad for your skin. The cult of oil-free moisturizers will have you believe oil causes acne. As a teenager, I totally bought into the oil-free, hypoallergenic, and noncomedogenic products. These products read like a barren wasteland of toxic ingredients. They don't contain oil, but they do contain lots of ingredients that strip your skin of moisture, leading to an overproduction of oil. Meaning, this stuff really doesn't work.

Our skin has sebaceous glands. They are located all over our body except on the palms of our hands and soles of our feet. Sebaceous glands produce sebum, which is the waxy oil that our body produces to keep our skin and hair moisturized. Talk about natural intelligence. Sebum is very close in its feel to jojoba oil, which is technically a wax not an oil. The oil on our skin isn't only sebum, but it is also made up of lipids from skin cells, sweat, and environmental matter.

When our skin doesn't produce enough sebum, our skin becomes dry. When it overproduces sebum, our skin gets oily. The key is to try to balance sebum production by balancing the oils on the face. Many oils, such as jojoba, can help us to find a healthy balance. Finding face and body oils that are right for you means knowing what your skin needs. It is most beneficial to apply oil to wet skin to both hydrate and moisturize.

Treating Dry Skin

Dry skin can be the result of not having enough fat (aka lipids) in the top layer of skin. Incorporate more omega-3s into your diet by eating more fresh fish (especially wild salmon), flaxseed oil, spinach, walnuts, and chia seeds. Look for products with heavier oils, such as jojoba, avocado, argan, and sea buckthorn, and butters, such as shea butter and cocoa butter. Wax such as beeswax and candelilla can help seal in moisture. Sea buckthorn oil can be used externally and internally to promote soft, supple skin.

Dry skin can also be caused by other factors such as dehydration, cold weather, dry weather, certain medications, and harsh detergents.

TONER, PH BALANCE & THE ACID MANTLE

Toner is one of those products that seems a bit mysterious. The words *pH balance* and *astringent* only make it more vague. So what does toner actually do and why is it important? Toner is traditionally applied after cleansing your skin to remove lingering makeup, dirt, pollution, and impurities. Use it before moisturizing, morning and night. Toner is also a perfect way to set mineral makeup and keep your skin looking dewy. Just spritz on your skin post makeup.

Toner also helps balance our pH levels. For a quick high school science refresh, pH stands for "potential of hydrogen" and measures the acidity of your skin. The measurement ranges from 1 to 14, 1 being highly acidic, 14 being alkaline, and 7 being neutral.

Our skin has a fine film on its surface called the *acid mantle*. It is slightly acidic and acts as a protective barrier, like a mantle or cloak. It keeps contaminants such as pollution, bacteria, and viruses from entering our skin. Sebum is secreted by the sebaceous glands and when mixed with sweat becomes the acid mantle.

The ideal pH for the face is slightly acidic, around 5.5. If your skin is prone to breakouts and oily, it is on the acidic side. If your skin is very dry, it is alkaline. The goal is to keep it balanced, and using a toner regularly, once or twice a day, helps find that sweet pH spot. Apple cider vinegar diluted at a 1-to-1 ratio with water is a great option for balancing skin.

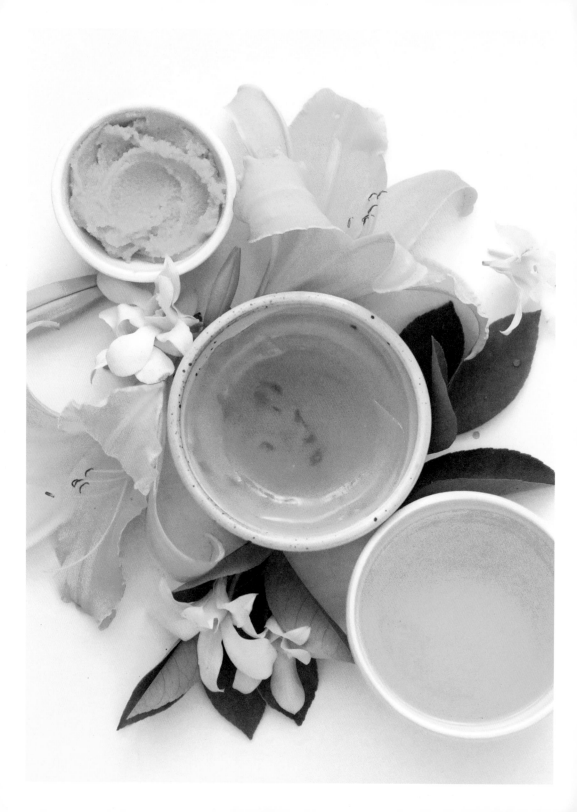

Toner can also be astringent, meaning it can shrink or tighten tissues, making your skin more taut and minimizing pores. Witch hazel is a perfect natural astringent that can be used directly on skin.

Using a hydrosol as a toner is a refreshing treat for your skin. Some hydrosols that are good for oily or acne-prone skin are peppermint, rosemary, tea tree, witch hazel, and rose geranium. For dry or combination skin, rose, lavender, frankincense, neroli, and chamomile are great options.

Collagen & Elastin

Collagen is the most common protein found in our bodies. It is integral to our connective tissues, forming the glue that holds everything together. Elastin is also a protein found in connective tissues. Both are integral to the health of our skin, even though they serve different functions. Elastin helps our skin retain its elasticity, helping it bounce back into shape after you stretch it. Collagen helps skin remain strong and firm. Our skin texture and shape is a result of collagen and elastin production. As we age, our bodies produce less of both proteins, leading to wrinkles, sagging skin, and slower wound healing. Collagen and elastin production can also be affected by poor diet and sun damage. We can naturally boost collagen production through eating vitamin C, making sure we get enough protein, and wearing sunscreen.

FREE RADICALS & ANTIOXIDANTS

"Free radicals" sounds like a rad band name, but they actually aren't the coolest things. They are naturally occurring molecules in our bodies that can cause oxidative stress, which causes cell damage throughout the body, including our skin. As we age, our body loses its ability to fight off free radicals, which can result in signs of aging such as wrinkles. We can accelerate the damage of free radicals in our body through overexposure to the sun; exposure to harsh chemicals, pollution, and pesticides; habits such as smoking and alcoholism; and a poor diet.

You have probably seen the words *free radical* and *antioxidants* used together. Antioxidants are molecules that can help us prevent the oxidative stress caused by free radicals. Many fruits, vegetables, legumes, and nuts are rich in antioxidants. Plant-based topical oils that contain antioxidants, such as vitamins A, C, and E, include rosehip seed oil and sea buckthorn oil.

BACTERIA & ACNE

Our skin and hair are covered in bacteria, which is a good thing. We have more than five hundred types of bacteria that form the skin's ecosystem, called a *microbiome*. Many of the bacteria are good, contributing to a healthy immune response. When the good bacteria are balanced and varied, our skin is clear and healthy. When the balance shifts, the bacteria can react. Acne is caused by a specific strain of bacteria called *Propionibacterium acnes*, which is present in all skin types. If our pores become clogged by not removing dead skin cells or if we strip our skin of its natural oils, it can become inflamed and erupt as a result. Gentle exfoliation several times per week with fine plant-based materials, like walnut powder, helps slough off dead skin cells; so do masks.

A bacterial imbalance is not just the result of external factors but internal ones as well. Our hormones and gut health contribute to the state of our skin's microbiome. Conventional over-the-counter topical treatments might kill bad bacteria, but they will wipe out the good bacteria as well. They will also dry out skin and cause other issues. Internal antibiotic treatments or more severe treatments such as Accutane can damage your gut health and lead to very serious side effects, which is why Accutane is now illegal in the United States.

Eating probiotics and foods high in zinc (e.g., pumpkin seeds and spinach), not overcleansing skin, sweating to help eliminate toxins, and creating an effective skin-care regime can be long-term solutions to clearer and healthier skin. Apple cider or witch hazel toners, gentle exfoliation, clay masks, gentle nondetergent cleansers, and essential oils such as antibacterial thyme, tea tree, and geranium are all powerful natural remedies. Also, stop touching your face all the time. I am as guilty of this as anyone else. Try to only touch your face with clean hands. Don't pick at it; treat it with care.

Acne is often caused by an imbalance of hormones. If you tend to break out around your period, this is most likely the cause. The main sex hormones in women are estrogen and progesterone. The two work in symphony to create a healthy hormone balance. Herbs and supplements can be used effectively to encourage balanced estrogen and progesterone production. Black cohosh (tincture or capsule) is used to balance estrogen production. Evening primrose oil (oil or capsule) and chaste tree (tincture or capsule) both work wonders for progesterone levels. Adding herbal adaptogens such as tulsi, ashwagandha, and maca into your daily routine is also a good idea because stress can alter progesterone production. Do not use any of these estrogen- and progesterone-balancing herbs if pregnant.

MIXING OIL & WATER

I recommend using oils or balms rather than moisturizers because conventional moisturizers can be mostly water. When water is added to any formula, manufacturers also add a strong preservative to keep the product from spoiling. Instead, I recommend making your own mix of oil and water.

If you apply face oil or body oil to moist skin after cleansing, you achieve the perfect balance of water and oil. Damp skin is more receptive to oil and helps seal in the moisture. You do not want to apply oil to dripping-wet skin. For the face, after cleansing or splashing your skin with warm or lukewarm water, lightly dry it and massage face oil into the skin. For the body, after bathing, lightly towel dry and apply body oil all over. This ritual is not only effective for soft, supple skin, but it is also delightful.

MOVING WITH THE SEASONS

In general, I think it is best to stick to your skin-care ritual and not change it too much each day, but I am a believer in adapting with the seasons. Just as you wouldn't reach for a hot soup on a sweltering day, your skin doesn't need a heavy face balm in the summer. Your skin care should move with the seasons, and, most of all, you should listen to what your face and body are craving. If your skin is dry and chapped, try a face balm that contains beeswax or a vegan plant-based wax to seal in moisture. Look for thicker body moisture with shea butter or cocoa butter to moisturize thirsty winter skin. In the summer, make sure to use toner regularly to effectively remove sweat and dirt. You can spritz yourself with hydrosol or toner throughout the day to maintain a fresh and cool feeling. Use a light oil or aloe to hydrate your body in warmer months. No matter what time of year, make sure to exfoliate your skin to slough off dead skin cells to prevent a bacterial imbalance.

SUNSHINE

Just like plants, we need the rays of the sun for our health and well-being. Our skin naturally produces and absorbs vitamin D when it is exposed to the sun. Vitamin D is known as the sunshine vitamin, and deficiency is very common. If you are feeling sluggish, this could be the culprit.

While the dangers of overexposure to the sun are well noted, we do need sunshine to thrive. You can eat foods rich in vitamin D, but there is so much pleasure to be gained from the feeling of sunshine on your body. Try to spend time outside every day for your well-being.

That said, damage from the sun can result in wrinkles, spots, and skin cancer. Wear mineral sunscreen with zinc and titanium dioxide instead of sunscreens that are full of harmful synthetic chemicals.

KISS & MAKEUP

Makeup is fun, really fun. What isn't fun are the ingredients in conventional brands. Lead, formaldehyde, coal tar dyes, and synthetic fragrance are but a few of the things that can easily end up painting our faces. Mica, the natural silicate mineral that adds luminosity to eye shadows and powders, is a contro-versial ingredient; unless it is certified as responsibly sourced, its mining may be linked to child labor.

If you wear lipstick, you inadvertently end up ingesting it. Additionally, heavy makeup can end up clogging our pores, especially if it isn't properly removed. All this is not to say don't wear makeup. I love makeup! Just look for brands that use plant-based ingredients and clean pigments. Make sure to remove makeup at night by cleansing your skin and using a gentle oil-based cleanser to remove eye makeup.

NAIL POLISH

Conventional nail polish contains a lot of terrifying ingredients, such as form-aldehyde. When you think about it, we are pretty much putting colored glue on our fingers and toes, so what are we expecting? If you use nail polish, look for formulas that are advertised as 9-free, meaning they don't include formal-dehyde, formaldehyde resin, toluene, DBP, camphor, xylene, ethyl tosylamide, parabens, and acetone.

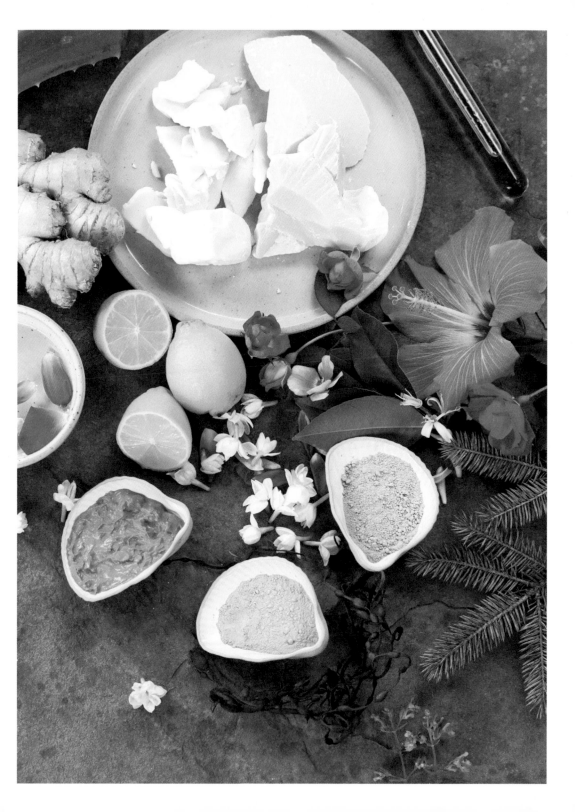

Cocoa & Spice Face Mask & Exfoliant

YIELD: 1½ OUNCES

INGREDIENTS

1 tablespoon bentonite clay
or kaolin clay

1 teaspoon activated
bamboo charcoal powder

1 tablespoon raw cocoa powder

1 teaspoon ground turmeric

¼ teaspoon ground nutmeg

¼ teaspoon ground cinnamon

¼ teaspoon ground ginger

ADDITIONAL EQUIPMENT

2-ounce glass jar with lid

This is a sumptuous mask and gentle exfoliant that I love in wintertime, but it is a great year-round treatment. It smells like spicy cocoa and soothes and clarifies skin without drying it out. Using activated charcoal and bentonite clay, which detoxify, along with antioxidant-rich raw cocoa powder and a potent blend of invigorating spices will leave your skin and senses feeling revived.

———————————————

Mix all ingredients together in small bowl. Pour into jar and close with lid. Will keep fresh for up to a year.

AS FACE MASK
Combine ½ teaspoon mix with ⅛ teaspoon water or hydrosol in small dish. Mix into paste and add more liquid if necessary for desired consistency. Apply to moist face and neck with fingers or brush. Leave on for 5 to 10 minutes, then rinse with lukewarm water. Pat dry with clean towel; apply toner and face oil or face balm.

AS EXFOLIANT
Apply quarter-size amount to wet face with fingers, massage gently into skin, and rinse with lukewarm water. Pat dry with clean towel; apply toner and face oil or face balm.

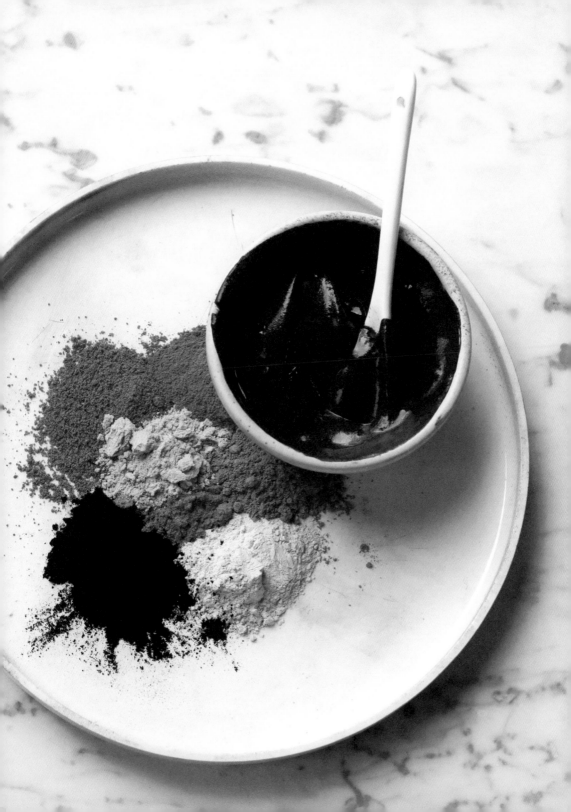

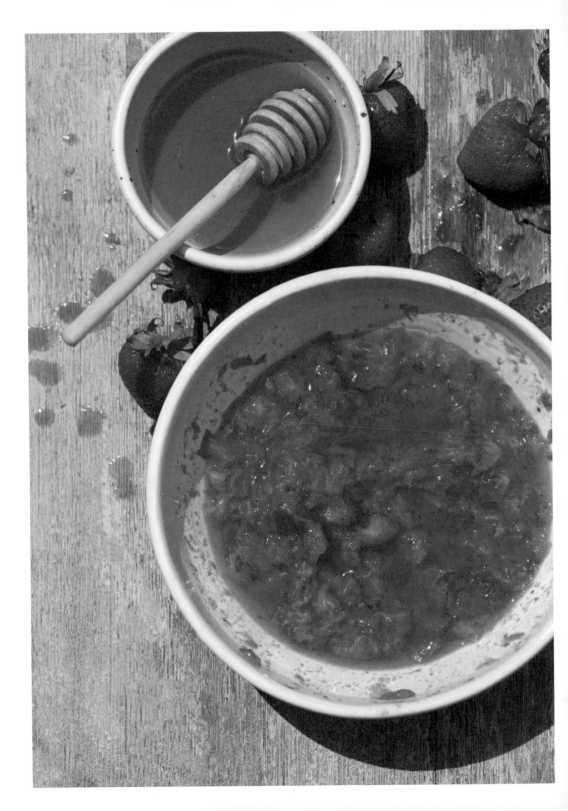

Fresh Face Fruit Mask

4 Variations

A simple fruit enzyme, yogurt, and honey mask brightens and rejuvenates skin year-round and is a real treat. It is easy to adapt to the seasons and the fresh fruit that you are eating that day. Make a little extra and eat it for breakfast or an afternoon snack.

Strawberry Soup Face Mask Inspired by my grandmother Milka's recipe.

Frutti di Bosco Face Mask I lived in Italy for a year and Frutti di Bosco, which means "fruits of the forest," was one of my favorite types of gelato.

Apple Crisp Face Mask The exfoliating malic acid in apples meets the spicy nutmeg for a powerful and mouth-watering encounter.

Peaches & Cream Face Mask Peaches are high in Vitamins A, C and E and antioxidants, which help improve skin health and texture.

Combine ingredients in small bowl. Wet face, pat dry. Apply mask to moist skin. Leave on for 10 to 20 minutes. Rinse off with lukewarm water.

**YIELD: ABOUT
1½ TABLESPOONS**

INGREDIENTS

1 teaspoon raw honey

1 tablespoon whole-milk yogurt, or soy or coconut yogurt

For Strawberry Soup Face Mask:

1 large strawberry, mashed

For Frutti di Bosco Face Mask:

1 raspberry, mashed

1 blackberry, mashed

2 blueberries, mashed

For Apple Crisp Face Mask:

¼ apple, mashed or blended in food processor

⅛ teaspoon ground nutmeg

For Peaches & Cream Face Mask:

½ peach, mashed

Maine Face Mask

YIELD: 1 TABLESPOON

INGREDIENTS

1½ teaspoons rose hydrosol

1 teaspoon French green clay

¼ teaspoon kelp powder

ADDITIONAL EQUIPMENT

Optional: mask brush

This detoxifying mask mixes purifying green clay, nourishing kelp, and soothing rosewater. It must be used immediately after making. Use once per week or as desired. Follow with toner and moisturizer of choice.

————————————————

Mix all ingredients together in small mixing bowl; stir well.

Apply immediately to moist face and neck with fingers or brush. Leave on for 5 to 10 minutes or until dry but not hardened. Remove with wet washcloth.

Clean Slate Makeup Remover & Oil-Based Cleanser

YIELD: 4 OUNCES

INGREDIENTS

¼ cup sunflower oil

2 tablespoons argan oil

2 tablespoons jojoba oil

½ teaspoon vitamin E

10 drops chamomile essential oil

10 drops lavender essential oil

ADDITIONAL EQUIPMENT

4-ounce glass bottle with pump

Using plant oils to remove makeup is not only effective but it is also incredibly soothing. What I love about this product is that it removes makeup and cleanses your skin while leaving it soft and supple. Use once or twice daily or as desired.

————————————————

Mix all ingredients together in measuring cup; stir well. Pour into glass bottle and attach pump.

Wet face and rub quarter-size amount of oil on face and around eyes. Remove with lukewarm water and wet washcloth. Follow with toner and cleanser of choice. If stored out of direct sunlight, will keep for up to a year

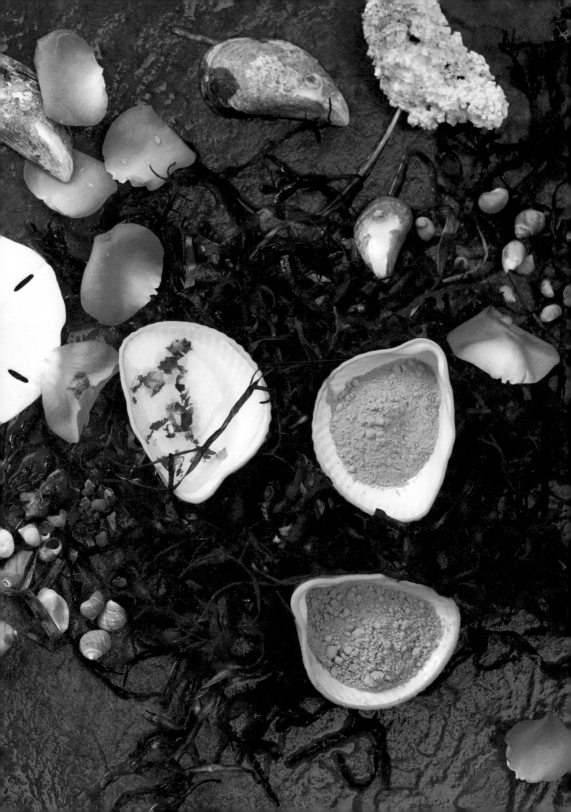

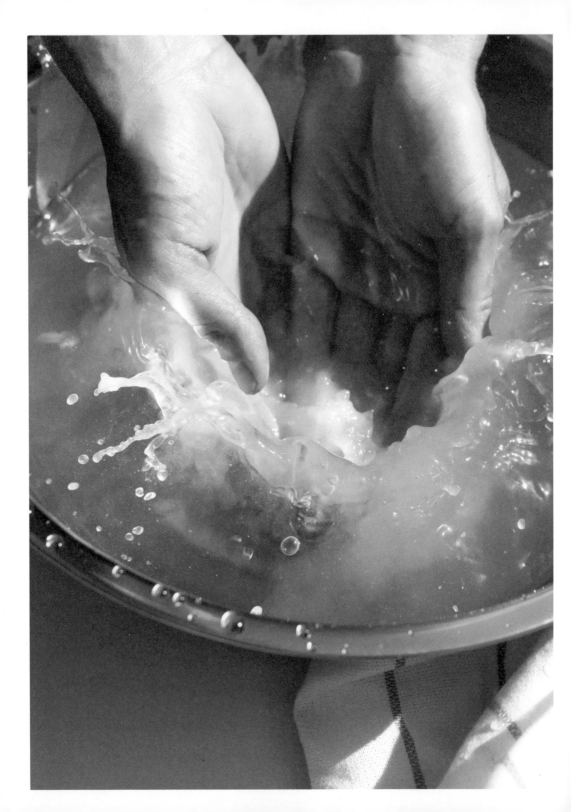

Creamy Shea Face Cleanser

I love a good cream cleanser, and this one doesn't disappoint. It cleanses skin without stripping it of moisture. The combination of shea butter, aloe, castile soap, and argan oil is a simple but powerful cocktail of ingredients. They create a gentle but effective wash that feels so rich and leaves skin so soft. Follow with toner and moisturizer of choice.

———————————————

Heat 1 to 2 inches of water in small pot over medium heat. Once it boils, turn down to simmer.

Add shea butter to measuring cup or jar and put in pot. Stir occasionally until fully melted, remove from heat. Wait until vessel is lukewarm to touch, and pour into mixing bowl with remaining ingredients. Use immersion blender to mix ingredients until creamy. Pour mixture into bottle and attach pump.

Use morning and night to cleanse face, or as desired. If stored out of direct sunlight, will keep for 6 months.

YIELD: 4 OUNCES

INGREDIENTS

2 tablespoons shea butter

⅓ cup aloe vera gel

2 tablespoons castile soap

1 tablespoon argan oil

½ teaspoon vitamin E

Optional: 5 drops lemongrass essential oil

ADDITIONAL EQUIPMENT

Immersion blender

4-ounce glass bottle with pump

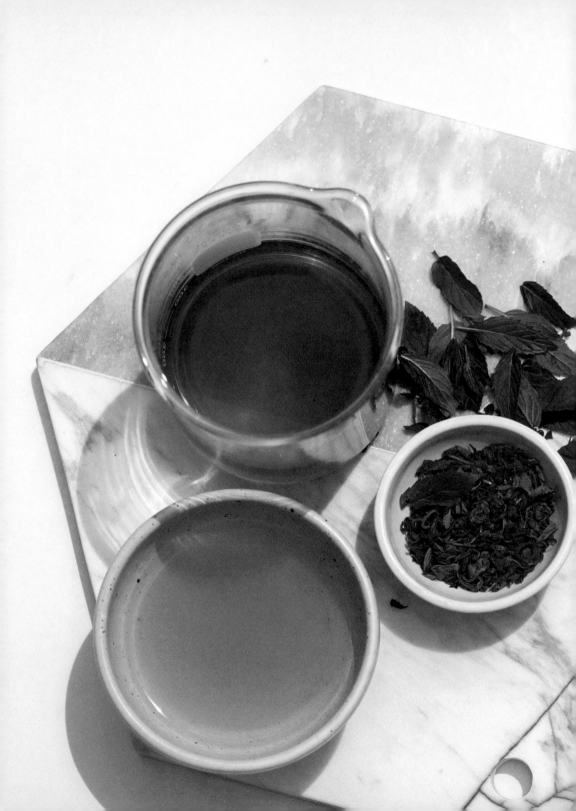

Fresh Green Tea Clarifying Toner

This toner is both cooling and clarifying, with anti-oxidant-rich green tea and astringent witch hazel, which is perfect for combination or oily skin. The invigorating mix of peppermint and tea tree essential oils helps soothe skin and prevent spots.

Combine all ingredients in measuring cup and stir well with spoon. Pour into bottle and attach sprayer.

Mist on face and pat in with fingers or cotton ball, or use as a refreshing body mist. Will keep for up to 3 months at room temperature, or store in fridge for up to 6 months.

YIELD: 4 OUNCES

INGREDIENTS

¼ cup green tea, cool

¼ cup witch hazel

5 drops peppermint essential oil

3 drops tea tree essential oil

Optional: 1 teaspoon apple cider vinegar

ADDITIONAL EQUIPMENT

8-ounce glass bottle, or two 4-ounce glass bottles, with fine-mist sprayer(s)

Smell the Roses Face Toner & Body Mist

YIELD: 8 OUNCES

INGREDIENTS

¾ cup witch hazel

¼ cup rose hydrosol

2 tablespoons aloe
vera gel or juice

Optional: 8 to 10 drops
rose essential oil*

ADDITIONAL EQUIPMENT

8-ounce glass bottle, or
two 4-ounce glass bottles,
with fine-mist sprayer(s)

* Add rose essential oil for
an even rosier scent if you
are a rose fanatic like me.

This refreshing mist helps hydrate and clarify skin and smells like a rose bush. It is perfect to put on skin to prime it for face oil. It is best kept in the fridge for freshness and is best enjoyed cold. It is also a great hair perfume and mist. Nothing is more invigorating than a spritz of cool rosy mist on your face, body, and hair on a hot summer day!

Combine all ingredients in large spouted measuring cup and stir well with spoon. Pour into bottle and attach sprayer.

Use morning and night on skin before moisturizer or during the day for a refreshing pick-me-up. Will keep at room temperature for up to 3 months, store in fridge for up to a year.

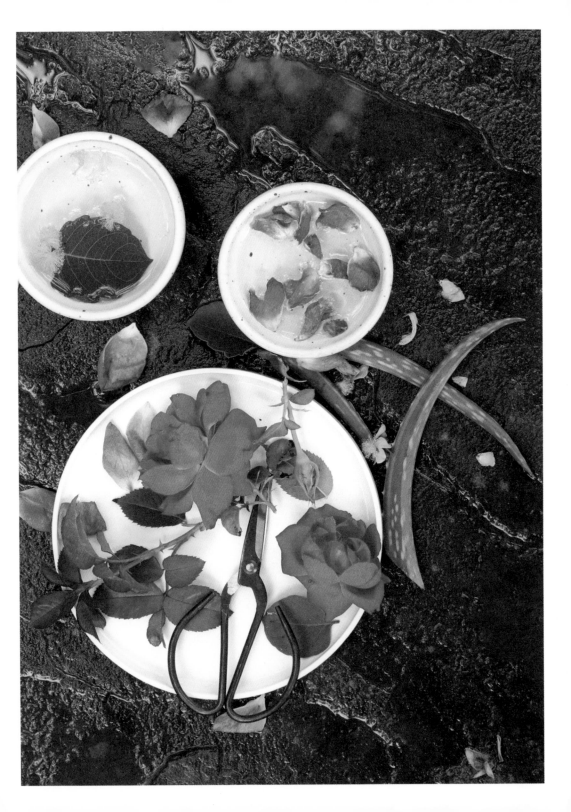

Golden Glow Face Balm

YIELD: 4 OUNCES

INGREDIENTS

¼ cup shea butter

2 tablespoons cocoa butter

1½ teaspoons beeswax or vegan wax

2 tablespoons jojoba oil

1 tablespoon rosehip seed oil

½ teaspoon vitamin E

⅛ teaspoon sea buckthorn oil

20 drops neroli or rose essential oil

ADDITIONAL EQUIPMENT

4-ounce glass jar with lid or two 2-ounce glass jars with lids

Don't get me wrong. I love face oil, but when my skin is chapped or very dry, I reach for face *balm*. This deeply nourishing balm is golden in feel and color, both sumptuous and decadent. Anti-inflammatory shea butter helps improve skin elasticity and firmness, while cocoa butter and wax seal in moisture. A full array of plant-carrier oils of jojoba, rosehip seed, and sea buckthorn add skin-nourishing vitamins and fatty acids. This soothing balm is great for chapped skin, inflamed skin, and eczema. I use this all winter long, but I love it anytime of year when I need deep moisture.

Heat 2 inches of water in small pot over medium heat. Once it boils, turn down to simmer.

Add shea butter, cocoa butter, and wax to measuring cup and put in pot. When fully melted, remove from heat. Wait until vessel is lukewarm to touch, and pour into mixing bowl with remaining ingredients. Stir well with spoon. Pour into jar with lid.

Use, with dry, clean fingers, morning and night as moisturizer or as needed. If stored out of direct sunlight, will keep for up to a year.

Deep Sleep Eye Serum

I know about puffy eyes, dark circles, and being weary; it is no fun. This refreshing balm can't offer you sleep, but it can help alleviate what lack of sleep does to your eyes. It soothes tired puffy eyes, nourishes dry skin, and prevents fine lines. I highly recommend keeping it in the fridge as it is delightful cold.

Heat 2 inches of water in small pot over medium heat. Once it boils, turn down to simmer.

Put shea butter in measuring cup and put in pot. When fully melted remove from heat. Wait until vessel is cool to touch, add remaining ingredients, and blend with immersion blender. Pour into jar with lid.

Use around eyes morning or night or as needed. Will keep for up to 6 months at room temperature, or store in fridge for up to a year.

YIELD: 2 OUNCES

INGREDIENTS

2 tablespoons shea butter

1 tablespoon aloe vera gel

1 tablespoon rosehip seed oil

½ teaspoon vitamin E

10 drops chamomile essential oil

5 drops frankincense essential oil

ADDITIONAL EQUIPMENT

Immersion blender

2-ounce glass jar with lid

Butterfly Daytime Face Oil

YIELD: 1 OUNCE

INGREDIENTS

2 tablespoons jojoba oil

1 tablespoon rosehip seed oil

5 drops jasmine, neroli, or
rose essential oil

ADDITIONAL EQUIPMENT

1-ounce glass bottle
with eyedropper

This is a simple but essential recipe for a daily face oil that you can use both morning and night all year-round. The combination of jojoba and rosehip seed oil is easily absorbed, helping to soothe inflamed skin, deliver rich moisture, remove dead skin cells, and unclog pores. Adding your favorite essential oil or extract to the mix makes the experience even more joyful. Jasmine, neroli, and rose, besides smelling amazing, help with skin rejuvenation.

Mix all ingredients together in measuring cup or bowl with metal spoon. Pour into bottle and close with eyedropper.

Use several drops on moist skin morning and night or as needed. If stored out of direct sunlight, will keep for up to a year.

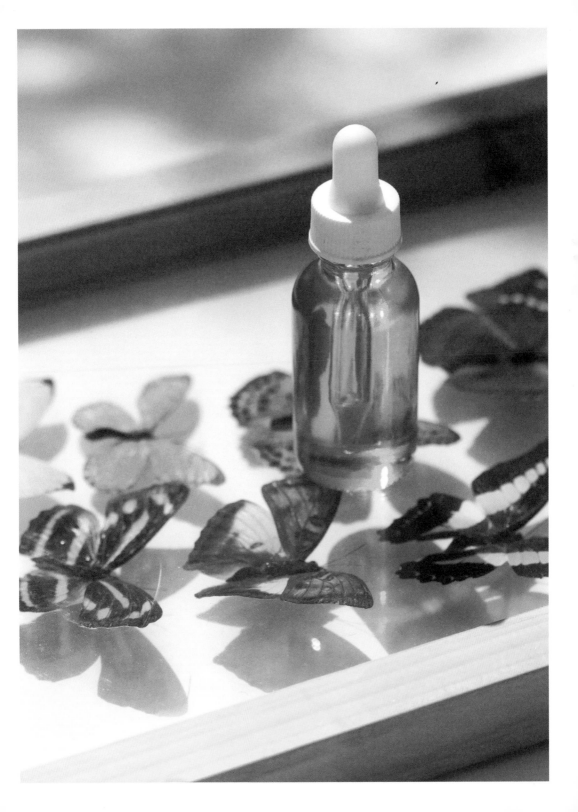

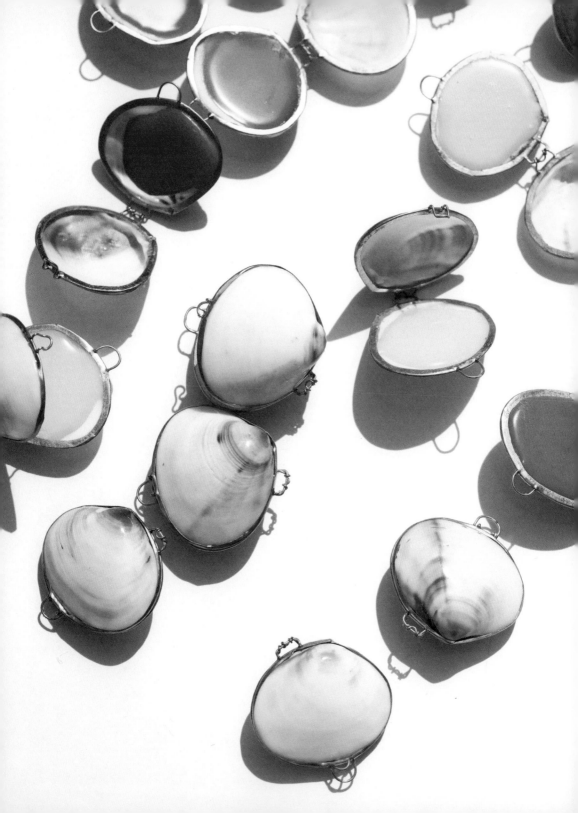

Lick Your Lips Balm

This sweet-smelling and -tasting balm combines luscious cocoa butter and coconut oil along with wax to seal in moisture. It is a real treat for parched lips any time of year. The two scent options give you a "Creamsicle" or mint chocolate treat; you can't go wrong. You can add alkanet root for a lightly tinted berry color (see variation).

Heat 2 inches of water in small pot over medium heat. When it boils, turn down to simmer.

Put cocoa butter, coconut oil, and wax in measuring cup and put in pot. When fully melted, remove from heat. Let mixture cool for several minutes and add vitamin E and essential oils of your choice. Stir well and pour into tin with lid. Let cool until fully hardened.

Apply with fingers to lips as desired. Will keep for up to a year.

VARIATION FOR COLORED BALM

If you use alkanet root (unpowdered), add 1 tablespoon to mixture while heating. After you remove from heat, strain with fine-mesh strainer to remove root.

If you use powdered alkanet root, add 1 teaspoon directly to mixture after you remove from heat and stir well.

YIELD: 1½ OUNCES

INGREDIENTS

2 tablespoons cocoa butter

2 tablespoons coconut oil

2 tablespoons beeswax or vegan wax

½ teaspoon vitamin E

For a creamsicle scent:

7 drops sweet orange essential oil

3 drops vanilla CO_2 extract

For a minty scent:

10 drops peppermint essential oil

Optional: 1 teaspoon alkanet root powder

ADDITIONAL EQUIPMENT

Metal tins with lids (either one 2-ounce tin or two 1-ounce tins or)

Shimmer & Pop Highlighter

YIELD: 1½ OUNCES

INGREDIENTS

2 tablespoons jojoba oil

1 tablespoon shea butter

1 tablespoon beeswax or
vegan wax

1 tablespoon mica
(silver, gold, or copper)

½ teaspoon vitamin E

ADDITIONAL EQUIPMENT

Metal tins with lids (either one
2-ounce tin or two 1-ounce tins)

If I want to make my eyes pop and add some shimmer to my face, I reach for a highlighter. This basic and easily adaptable recipe will allow you to make an array of different highlighters for your skin. I like to put it around my eyes and on my cheekbones. You can choose any color of mica you want, but silver, copper, and gold make for subtle shimmer and shine. Always make sure you buy natural and responsibly sourced mica.

————————————

Heat 2 inches of water in small pot over medium heat. When it boils, turn down to simmer.

Add jojoba oil, shea butter, and wax to measuring cup and put in pot. When fully melted, remove from heat. Let mixture cool for several minutes and add mica and vitamin E. Stir well and pour into tin. Put on lid and let cool until fully hardened.

Apply with fingers or brush around eyes and cheeks or as desired. Will keep for up to a year.

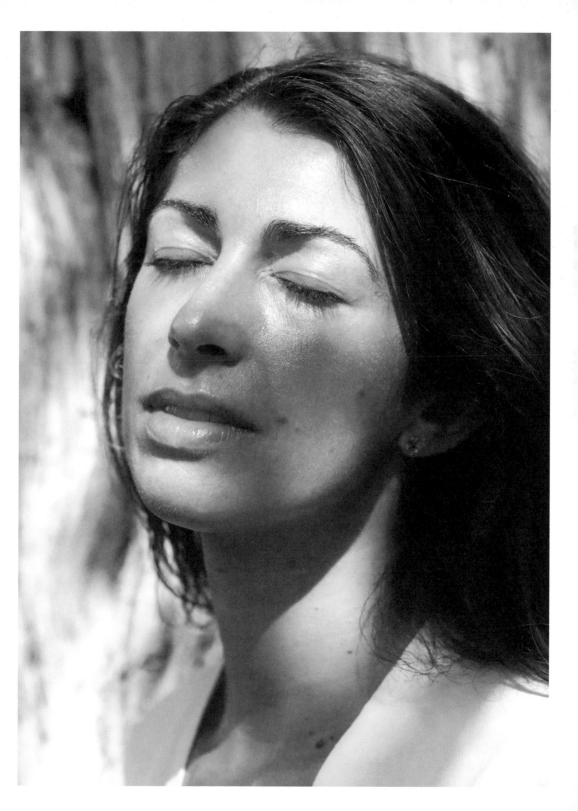

CHAPTER FIVE

Hair

Symbolic of life, hair bolts from our head[s]. Like the earth, it can be harvested, but it will rise again. We can change its color and texture when the mood strikes us, but in time it will return to its original form. . . ."[13]

Diane Ackerman, *A Natural History of the Senses*

While people often take good care of their skin, they treat their hair with reckless abandon. Overwashing and using harsh chemicals, dyes, and heat tools can ravage your scalp and your hair, leading to itchy scalp, dandruff, hair breakage, and hair loss. Each strand of our hair is made of the protein keratin, which connects to our skin through a hair follicle. Tiny blood vessels in our scalp deliver nutrients to the follicles to keep our hair healthy. Hair follicles cover all of our skin, except on our palms and the soles of our feet. It is one of the defining characteristics of mammals.

Instead of overwashing and using harsh shampoos, styling products, dyes, and heat tools, I suggest a gentler approach. Try to wash your hair only once or twice a week with a natural sulfate-free shampoo and conditioner. Blow-dry as little as possible. Air-dry your hair or get yourself a natural-fiber hair towel. You can wet your hair in between washes and use conditioner, or I highly recommend using dry shampoo.

Just as our skin has a microbiome, or ecosystem, so does our scalp. When we use harsh detergent shampoos on our hair, we end up damaging that microbiome. Dandruff has been linked to an imbalance of bacteria in our microbiome. Apple cider vinegar rinses can help restore scalp health through balancing pH and removing product buildup. Regular scalp massages with oil are a delight for the senses and for the health of the scalp. The key to luscious hair is treating it lusciously.

Taking Care of Hair

STYLE

Conventional hair-styling products are often toxic. Most hair sprays, hair gels, and mousses include ingredients such as ethanol, parabens, butane, hydrochlorofluorocarbon, and butylene glycol.

Great natural alternative styling products include sea-salt hair sprays, gels rich with aloe vera, and styling waxes with plant-based butters and waxes.

DRY SHAMPOO

I live by dry shampoo. I wash my hair once or twice a week max and use dry shampoo to freshen it between washes. Powdered dry shampoos absorb oil, mask grease, and add volume. Watch out for aerosol dry shampoos that contain toxic ingredients, like butane.

GOOD OILS

I cannot sing the praises of hair oil highly enough. Just like face oil, hair oil is a secret weapon. To replenish dry hair and add luster, a hair oil rich in light plant-based oils such as argan, jojoba, sunflower, and camellia seed is a must. It can be rubbed into the ends of dry hair for an instant thirst quench. Hair oil can be massaged into the scalp and all over the hair for a deeper treatment that can be done weekly or as needed. It also helps define hair and tame frizz.

EXFOLIATE & MASK

Like your face, your scalp benefits from exfoliation, which helps remove product buildup and sloughs off dead skin cells. I recommend adding a tablespoon of fine sugar or sea salt to your shampoo at least twice a month, rubbing it into your scalp and rinsing. Just like a mask for your skin, a hair mask gently exfoliates and draws out toxins, leaving hair soft and clean.

DYE

As a teenager, I had a rainbow of hair colors on my head. I haven't dyed my hair since then, but I remember it was fun. Honestly, most hair dyes are really toxic for your body and not good for your hair.

Now there are more natural hair-coloring products using safer ingredients. Do your research before coloring your hair, or choose to go au naturel.

BRUSHING

Brushing your hair is a beautiful and soothing ritual. It helps spread the natural oils from your scalp throughout your hair. Always use a natural-bristle brush or wooden comb. Plastic bristles or combs can hurt your scalp and damage your hair, leading to breakage.

Mermaid Hair Mask

YIELD: 2 OUNCES

INGREDIENTS

1 tablespoon kelp powder

1 tablespoon bentonite clay
or kaolin clay

¼ cup water or cooled nettle tea

1 teaspoon apple cider vinegar

I am not gonna lie; this smells briny like the ocean. It makes me feel like I am on the beach smelling seaweed drying in the sun. This gently exfoliating and detoxifying blend with bentonite clay and seaweed cleanses environmental elements, such as dirt and pollution, and rejuvenates your hair and scalp. Apple cider vinegar removes buildup, balances scalp pH, and adds shine. This mask leaves hair clean, soft, and shiny. Use twice a month or as desired. Follow with Milk & Honey Shampoo (page 122) and Witchy Coconut Leave-In Conditioner & Detangler (page 126).

Add kelp and clay to small mixing dish and mix with spoon. Add water and vinegar and stir to form paste.

Apply paste to damp hair with fingers, rubbing into scalp and all the way down to ends of hair. Leave on for 15 minutes. Rinse with warm water until water runs clear.

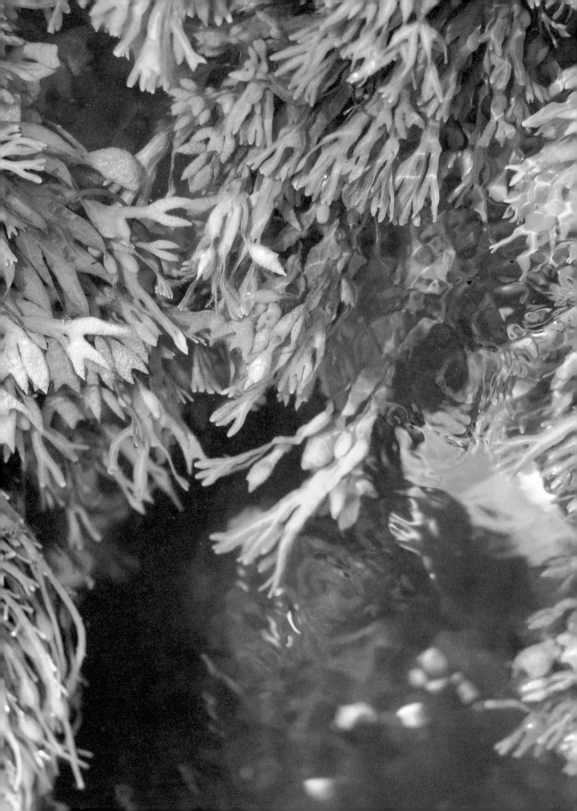

Milk & Honey Shampoo

YIELD: ABOUT 6 OUNCES

INGREDIENTS

¼ cup simple coconut milk*

¼ cup rose hydrosol

1 tablespoon raw honey

¼ cup castile soap**

* Choose a full-fat coconut milk that doesn't have any additives.

** You might want to increase or decrease amount of castile soap depending on what works best with your hair. It might take a few washes for your hair to adjust to this gentle shampoo.

ADDITIONAL EQUIPMENT

Immersion blender

6- to 8-ounce glass bottle with lid

This is a gentle but effective shampoo with four superstar ingredients. Castile soap cleanses, coconut milk moisturizes, rose hydrosol aids scalp health and hair growth, and honey helps strengthen hair. Follow with Refreshing Hibiscus ACV Rinse (facing page).

Combine coconut milk, rose hydrosol, and honey in small bowl and blend together with immersion blender for 10 seconds. Add castile soap and stir with spoon. Pour into bottle with lid.

Use once or twice weekly or as desired. Will keep for up to 1 month at room temperature, or store in fridge for up to 6 months.

Refreshing Hibiscus ACV Rinse

Using castile soap in your hair is an effective cleanser, but it can throw off the pH of your scalp because it is very alkaline. This acidic hair rinse will restore pH, remove soap residue, and leave your hair soft and shiny. It is perfect to use after Milk & Honey Shampoo (facing page). Aloe vera gel soothes the scalp and nourishes hair. Hibiscus not only provides a beautiful hue to this rinse, but it is also a superpower ingredient to promote hair growth. Follow with Witchy Coconut Leave-In Conditioner & Detangler (page 126).

YIELD: 16 OUNCES

INGREDIENTS

2 teaspoons dried hibiscus flowers*

1 cup aloe vera gel

¼ cup apple cider vinegar

* Can also alternate with nettle or chamomile tea for variety.

ADDITIONAL EQUIPMENT

16-ounce bottle with lid

Heat 1 cup water in small pot over medium heat. When it boils steep hibiscus flowers for 10 minutes. Strain and set liquid aside to cool in small mixing bowl. Once liquid is cool, add remaining ingredients and stir with spoon. Pour into bottle with lid. Store in fridge for up to 1 month.

To apply to hair, pour ½ cup in small bowl and then pour over just-shampooed hair, rubbing into scalp and throughout ends. Leave on for at least 1 minute and then rinse well.

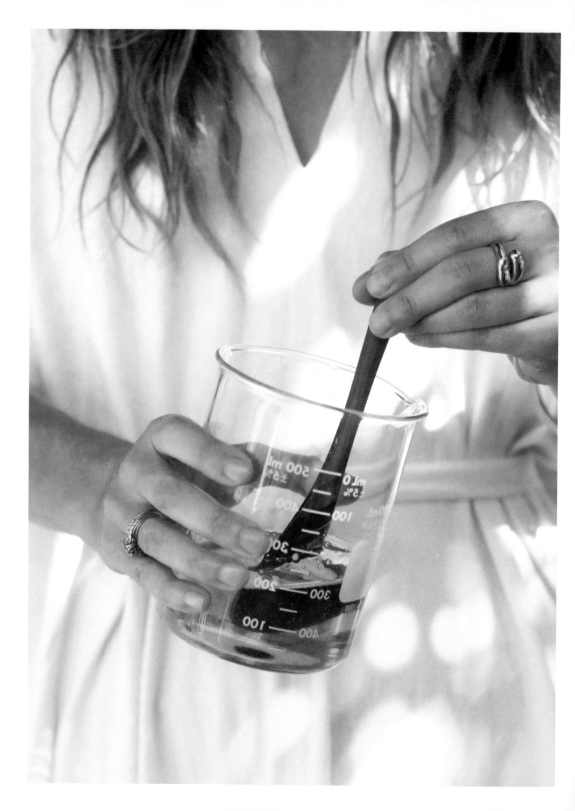

Shining Waves Hair Oil

Just like face oil, this hair oil imparts moisture and glow. It instantly adds shine and prevents frizz and flyaways. This potent blend of hair-nourishing carrier oils and essential oils will bring life and softness to your mane.

———————————

Combine all ingredients in measuring cup and stir with spoon. With funnel, pour into glass bottle and close with eyedropper.

Use on wet or dry hair or as needed. If stored out of direct sunlight, will keep for up to 2 years.

YIELD: 1 OUNCE

INGREDIENTS

2 tablespoons argan oil

1 tablespoon jojoba oil

5 drops rosemary essential oil

5 drops ylang ylang essential oil

2 drops lavender essential oil

Optional: ⅛ teaspoon
sea buckthorn oil

ADDITIONAL EQUIPMENT

Small metal funnel

1-ounce glass bottle
with eyedropper

Sea Salt Wave Spray

YIELD: 4 OUNCES

INGREDIENTS

½ cup distilled water

1 tablespoon sea salt

1 tablespoon aloe vera gel

10 drops lemongrass or lavender essential oil

Optional: ½ teaspoon argan oil for moisture

ADDITIONAL EQUIPMENT

4-ounce spray bottle with fine-mist sprayer

For textured hair all year-round, this is my go-to. A mix of this and Sail-Away Dry Shampoo (facing page) is all I need each day. A simple but effective blend to give you that just-left-the-beach look without leaving your hair crunchy.

───────────────

Heat water in small pot over medium heat. When it boils, remove from heat, add sea salt, and stir until dissolved. Let mixture cool thoroughly. Add aloe vera gel, essential oil, and argan (if using) and stir. Pour into bottle.

Spray in hair, scrunch, and style for texture. Reapply as often as necessary. If stored out of direct sunlight, will keep for up to a year.

Witchy Coconut Leave-In Conditioner & Detangler

YIELD: 4 OUNCES

INGREDIENTS

¼ cup witch hazel

¼ cup simple coconut milk*

* Choose a full-fat coconut milk that doesn't have any additives.

This simple but delicious recipe helps condition and detangle your hair and smells like a tropical milkshake. Coconut milk helps restore and revive dry, damaged hair and helps prevent split ends.

───────────────

Mix all ingredients together in a measuring cup and stir well. Pour into bottle and attach sprayer. Mixture may separate; shake well before use.

Use on wet hair or on dry hair for added moisture. If stored in refrigerator, will keep for up to 6 months.

Sail-Away Dry Shampoo

An easy, breezy dry shampoo to sprinkle in your hair, rub in, and sail on with your day. This simple recipe will become a staple in your routine and make shampooing less frequent. It masks grease and adds body to second-, third-, fourth- (you get it) day hair. This fine powder blends easily into all hair colors, but you can add cocoa powder to create a brunette shade that blends into brown or black hair. You can blend with fingers or with a hairbrush or a quick blast of a blow dryer.

Mix all ingredients together in measuring cup. With funnel, pour into shaker, or spoon into container. Close with lid.

Sprinkle generously onto your roots and rub in with fingers. Use in the morning, after working out, or as necessary for a quick refresh. Will keep for up to 2 years.

YIELD: 8 OUNCES

INGREDIENTS

½ cup arrowroot powder or cornstarch

2 tablespoons bentonite or kaolin clay

1 tablespoon baking soda

Optional: ¼ cup raw cocoa powder

30 drops lavender or lemongrass essential oil

ADDITIONAL EQUIPMENT

Small metal funnel

Shaker container, glass with metal lid, or repurposed salt or spice shaker

CHAPTER SIX

Wild Nature

"When the chesty, fierce-furred bear becomes sick he travels the mountainsides and the fields, searching for certain grasses, flowers, leaves, and herbs that hold within themselves the power of healing. He eats, he grows stronger. Could you, oh clever one, do this?"[14]

Mary Oliver, *Upstream*

*E*very time we have moved in the past ten years, my cat Siga has gotten lost. She always comes back or we find her, but I feel like it is her taking her time to get her bearings on her new home. I am like my cat when it comes to change. When I moved from the San Francisco Bay Area to a town of four hundred in the Hudson River Valley, I was initially elated to be in the country, but then I became totally unanchored. It took a year for me to start feeling at home. I spent time hiking in the mountains by our new home as my daughter grew in my belly. I got to know the landscape, found the swimming spots, and learned the native plants. I got my bearings physically, emotionally, and mentally and then I really started to grow here.

One of the first plants I learned about when I moved to our area was jewel-weed (*Impatiens capensis*). After getting a nasty swath of poison ivy on my leg, I learned about this plant revered by Native Americans as a natural antidote. Jewelweed, so named since its leaves turn iridescent silver when immersed in water, can be used to soothe and heal poison ivy. It tends to grow alongside poison ivy, meaning the poison and its remedy intermingle. The intelligence of wild nature is profound and is something we have a lot to learn from.

I began to study herbalism near my home with the amazing Dina Falconi, who is an herbalist, teacher, author, and activist. In our class that unfolded with the growing season, we learned to identify plants in Dina's extraordinary garden. Unlike most gardens, hers is an intentional mix of cultivated and wild plants. We learned their many uses. Did you know that Queen Anne's lace, also known as wild carrot, is made into a precious carrier oil with a natural SPF and that its seeds are used as a natural form of birth control (don't try this at home)? Falconi writes that "to forage means to dance with the land."[15] By coexisting with the wild and the cultivated, we can have a foot in two worlds.

Many medicinal and edible plants grow right outside our doors—even in cities!—but we have forgotten their names and their powers. As I gaze out my window at the field in front of my house, I see red clover, dandelion, dame's rocket, yellow dock, burdock root, and one plant to kindly respect and avoid, poison ivy. I also see the sweet briar rose, a favorite of Shakespeare's, which was first cultivated in Europe in the sixteenth century. The rambling rose now runs through fields of ferns and climbs up trees perfuming our town every June with its sweet dappled rose-and-apple scent. Learning about these plants—their names, characteristics, smells, and uses—it is impossible not to cultivate a deep reverence for nature.

Plant medicine, or herbalism, is the oldest medicine. Ancient wisdom involving the use of plants for self-care, both internally and externally, has been passed down from generation to generation. Meanwhile, secrets have been uncovered and rediscovered. Herbalism treats the whole person not just the symptoms, because everything is interconnected. However, living in balance with our bodies and listening to their desires is not always easy. The busyness of life can wash over us in waves, and it is easy to get swept away and go adrift. We have only this one body, and it is important to honor it and treat it with respect. This is easier said than done. What we put in our bodies, our habits, our state of mind, is a reflection of our well-being. There is so much that is out of our control in the world, but what we can control is how we treat ourselves and others, hopefully with love, kindness, compassion, and wonder.

When we bought our house, people kept telling us how lucky we were to have Old Ford Farm at the end of our road. I didn't know what that was at the time, but I have been continually delighted since I found out. It is an incredible honor-system farm run by a young family and is open twenty-four hours a day. Within a short walk, we have access to raw organic milk, eggs, vegetables, and many other fresh local products. It is hard to deny the delight of the taste of the first strawberry of the season or a sun-ripened cherry tomato picked off the vine. Not to mention the aromatic delight and depth of basil or cilantro. We have such a rich palette of natural tastes to work with, it seems crazy that synthetic flavors are added to "enhance" food.

Food is fuel for our bodies, but it is also medicine. Food can be nourishing, healing, and pleasurable. In my opinion, just like beauty products, food is best when the ingredients are simple but full of integrity. In this chapter, I want to share with you some of my personal anecdotes for finding balance with my mind and body, wonder in nature, and some simple recipes for plant-based teas and elixirs for skin and body.

Self Care

This spring I took the time to travel with friends to the desert and dip into hot springs. After a long bout with the flu, taking a window away from the world to focus on self-care was the best medicine. I tend to run fast and treat myself like a human pinball machine. I am passionate and want life to be full, but time and again, I keep relearning that less is more. My mother has told me, since I was a child, that I needed to find freedom through discipline. It's my mantra that I keep coming back to. I try to assert anchors in my days to keep myself afloat.

Taking time for self-care is and isn't easy. While you're aware of your body's quirks—its rashes, its aches—prioritizing the care of the whole self can be hard. Maybe it is establishing a ritual such as self-care Sunday or just taking five or ten minutes to meditate each day. Even if brief, taking time for yourself is a powerful practice with deep benefits. I find my best ideas and inspiration come when I give myself a break. Most weeks, running or walking with my dog each day is my ritual to get the time and space to expand. Or when I get a bit of extra time, I go to the mountains and hike to my sacred spot, a waterfall in the woods. This is a place I have returned to often throughout the seasons, a place that gives me reinforcement, perspective, and a sense of peace.

I am someone who loves my meditation practice and then abandons it for a year. I crave ritual in my life but easily fall out of it. Recently, I have started meditating again every morning. Instead of a "perfect" practice, chirping children or a cat rubbing up against me is the norm. I fall out of focus and then back in. I have realized that this is life. Instead of giving up, we have to learn how to roll with the tides and stay balanced throughout. It means embracing the perfect imperfect. Even if it's just one minute of being silent and focusing on breathing, it can change your outlook on the day. The most important thing is just to be.

WILD NATURE

"The wild nature has a vast integrity to it."[16]
CLARISSA PINKOLA ESTÉS

Mandy Aftel told me to read Clarissa Pinkola Estés's *Women Who Run with the Wolves*, and I am so grateful. It was a book I saw on my mom's bookshelf growing up and one that I have wanted to read for ages. I think things find you at the right time in your life. This book was definitely seminal in a lot of my thinking for my book, especially the narratives around wild nature, wild beauty, and wild women. Estés writes that wild nature means:

". . . to establish one's territory, to find one's pack, to be in one's body with certainty and pride regardless of the body's gifts and limitations, to speak and act in one's behalf, to be aware, alert, to draw on the innate feminine powers of intuition and sensing, to come into one's cycles, to find what one belongs to, to rise with dignity, to retain as much consciousness as possible."[17]

This description seems like ancient knowledge passed down from a great-grandmother, the simple but resounding cry to dig your feet in, find yourself, trust yourself, deeply connect with your kindred family, and be as fully aware as possible.

Wild beauty is an expression of wild nature. It means achieving beauty naturally inside and out. To know that there is not one way to be or to live. Our intuitive path is the way that works for us. One of my favorite things to do is take a walk down our street with my dog under the full moon. I walk guided by the light of the moon and know this road like the back of my hand. My two eyes, my dog's two eyes, the many other eyes lighting the night, my steps landing as they should, I always feel aware and connected to something larger, a breathing universe full of stars.

Gratitude

Lately my daughter, Mila, wakes up singing in the morning. Sometimes it is before 6 a.m., and I just want to go back to sleep, yet I can't help but smile at the sweetness of the songs she is making up as she goes. Often my son and daughter chase each other around the house in circles screaming, and it gets irritating but it is also joyful. I have been hanging close to these moments, trying to appreciate them and realizing one day how much I will miss them. I know that in no time Mila will be thirty-seven, like I am as I write this book, and, hopefully, I will be telling her these stories.

I wrote this book while grappling with two terminal illnesses in my family. It tends to only be in these moments of hardship that we realize the abundance of what we have in our lives. The wild life that courses through our veins is so precious, as are the experiences we get to share with those we love. It is in these times that we wish we had a magic wand to change reality, but instead the magic really is the time we have together and the beauty and love that surrounds us. In seemingly mundane everyday rituals, you might even find some magic. Today, I took a run with my dog and was swept away by the sweet smell of the wild honeysuckle bushes wafting throughout the neighborhood. Just those minutes relishing in the smells colored my day.

As I grow my family and my business at the base of the Shawangunk Mountains, my roots go deeper with each year. Finding balance is always a process but one I am conscious of. We are happiest when we are connected and in tune with ourselves, our surroundings, and the ones we love. Wild beauty is an appeal to the senses and an appeal to freedom, desire, and wonder. It is keeping your eyes open to intuition. Wild nature is not only growing outside but inside us. Have you ever seen what mint can do in a garden? It takes root and runs. With intention, I believe we can all manifest like mint. Pick some mint, make some tea, and drink to that.

EAT
Try to eat as freshly as you can. Avoid prepackaged foods if you can. Choose organic and local when possible. If you eat meat, know exactly where it comes from. Make it a ritual to go to the farmers' market or join a CSA (Community Supporting Agriculture program), giving residents access to regional produce. Eat colorfully, and take pleasure in the taste, smell, and delight of food.

Cultivate your gut health by eating probiotics. Drink kombucha, eat yogurt, use vinegar in your salads, and add sauerkraut to them. My grandmother Milka used to make "strawberry soup" for us when we were kids, and it is a recipe I now make for my kids and myself. It is whole milk yogurt (or vegan yogurt), sliced strawberries, and honey (or maple syrup) to taste; mix well and enjoy.

DRINK

Consume water. Lots of it. It is so easy to get dehydrated, which ends up making you feel tired and depleted. If you want to liven it up, try the Mer-Made Energy Drink recipe (page 143), make iced herbal tea, or simply add alkalizing lemon juice to your water. Buy a good water filter for your house; it is well worth it, and you will drink more water as a result of it.

I love a good cup of coffee in the morning and fine wine, like anyone else. The key is not overdoing it and taking breaks. If you drink caffeine, make sure to follow that cup of tea or coffee with a glass of water. Try to limit your coffee to one cup per day, and, if you need an afternoon boost, try adding maca root to your smoothie or having a cup of green or black tea.

MOVE

When I lived in California, I took classes with incredible dancer Anna Halprin. Her classes are very much centered on finding your own expression through your body, making it up as you go. Her advice is to "do a little dance every day." No matter how much energy you have, what mood you are in, or what the weather is, try to move your body every day for at least half an hour. Try walking, hiking, swimming, dancing, surfing, yoga, or any other form of movement, whatever you desire. Exercise in moderation positively affects our whole being. We eat better, sleep better, and are more relaxed. Plus, sweating is actually good for your skin as it releases toxins.

CREATE

I once had a crabby art professor in college who told our class that we should just look at artwork by artists we liked and copy it. I couldn't think of anything more dispiriting to say to a young artist, as if there weren't enough beauty, creativity, and inspiration to go around. Instead I say look to those whom you admire, examine why you respect them, and find your own way. No one can make magic quite like you. You reflect and create beauty in your own way.

CRYSTALS

As a child, I was obsessed with my rock collection. When we moved to the base of the Shawangunk Mountains in the Hudson Valley, I had no idea crystal veins ran through this land or that water-clear Herkimer diamonds could be found close by. Right before my daughter, Mila, was born, I found my first crystals, and since then, hunting for them has become one of my favorite activities. To be able to find crystals near my home is a real gift. Clear quartz crystals are believed to have the power to clear negative energy and help promote focus, harmony, and balance. They also have the ability to collect energy, both positive and negative, and I suggest cleansing and charging them energetically. First, clean your crystals of any dirt and debris with a toothbrush if necessary. Then let them soak in a metal or glass bowl filled with seawater or homemade salt water for up to a week. I also suggest letting them bathe outside in the light of a full moon to cleanse and charge them every month or as often as possible.

The crystal industry is booming, but at what cost? Like the mica industry, it can be a very murky place. Just like "blood diamonds," crystals can come at the cost of the exploitation of natural resources and child labor, plus the resulting violence. This seems to negate the positive qualities of a stone. It is important to know the provenance of your crystals. If you are purchasing stones, ask the seller where the crystal came from, how it was harvested and acquired. Knowing the story of a crystal only makes it a more powerful ally for you. And, you never know, maybe there are crystals growing near your home, too.

SLEEP

Take it from a mama with two young ones: I know it is hard to get enough sleep. For me, it sometimes means sleeping in my daughter's twin bed with her through the night. It is important to make sleep a priority. When we don't get enough, every part of our being suffers, as do the loved ones who have to deal with our cranky selves. Try to create a ritual around bedtime to signal to your senses it is time for dreams. Maybe it is drinking a calming tea, spritzing your pillows with a room spray, or using the same balm on your hands and feet every night.

Herbal Allies & Medicinal Foods

Probiotics are naturally occurring bacteria and yeast that are good for your health, especially your gut health. Foods such as yogurt, sauerkraut, pickles, kombucha, and, ahem, even dark chocolate are all probiotic foods.

Adaptogens are plants that support our reaction to stress. They are beneficial to our nervous and endocrine systems. Adaptogens have different characteristics; some are stimulating (maca, schizandra, and ginseng) and some are calming (tulsi), but generally these plants help with stress and related nervousness and anxiety. Other adaptogenic plants include ashwagandha, astragalus, cordyceps, and rhodiola.

Immune-boosting plants can help strengthen and support our ability to ward off illness. Some common ones I like to use when I am feeling run down or feel a cold coming on are cat's claw, echinacea, oregano, thyme, bee balm (great fresh in salads), ginger, mushrooms (such as reishi, chaga, shiitake, maitake), astragalus, and elderberry. Elderberry syrup is an integral part of a winter immune-system kit.

Cleansing herbs help us support the organs that filter toxins from our bodies. We just need to look to our skin to see how our system is functioning. When healthy, our skin is toned, smooth, and hydrated. Imbalances can manifest on our skin as acne, eczema, or rashes. The liver works tirelessly to detoxify our blood before it flows to the rest of our body. If it is not functioning properly, we fall out of balance. Getting enough sleep, managing stress, eating well, refraining from smoking, and monitoring caffeine and alcohol can help our liver function properly. Yet, other organs such as our lymph system and colon are also integral to our body's detoxification. Cleansing herbs can help. Examples include red clover, dandelion, burdock, yellow dock, red root, and nettle.

Digestive plants, or carminatives, aid with digestion, gas, and bloating. To improve digestion, peppermint, chamomile, fennel, ginger, cardamom, anise, cinnamon, and licorice root are perfect for teas and tinctures. Drinking a mug of ginger, chamomile, or peppermint tea after a meal helps to soothe your tummy.

Memory herbs are powerful for stimulating focus and improving cognition. Herbs such as gotu kola, ginseng, gingko, lemon balm, rosemary, peppermint, spearmint, and rhodiola are powerful allies. Another aid is regularly drinking antioxidant-rich green tea.

Women's health herbs can help us to nourish our bodies and connect with our cycles. A traditional tea for fertility and during pregnancy combines nettle, raspberry leaf, and oatstraw. This is a perfect tea for any time in our lives, as it is high in beneficial minerals and vitamins. Just red raspberry leaf alone is full of calcium, iron, and vitamins A, B, C, and E. This powerhouse of a tea helps strengthen bones, reduce inflammation, and support uterine health, helping to regulate menstruation. It also calms the nervous system, aids the endocrine system, and helps the adrenal system.

Other herbs that can help with women's hormonal support by balancing estrogen and progesterone production are vitex, damiana, black cohosh, and red clover.

Skin-care herbs help promote the health of our largest organ and address particular conditions, both internally and externally. For conditions such as dry skin or eczema, a tea with detoxifying and anti-inflammatory herbs such as tulsi, nettle, lemon balm, and red clover can help. For acne, a tea with turmeric, ginger, dandelion, yellow dock, and burdock can help restore balance and proper body function.

Dried lavender, rose, chamomile, plantain, comfrey, and calendula can be infused in oil for an all-purpose soothing skin oil.

Your Sanctuary

Our home is our sacred space, a place for respite and joy. Treat your home and belongings with respect just as you would your body. When we use synthetic chemicals to clean our homes, clothing, dishes, and belongings, we end up affecting the health of ourselves, our families, and our pets.

It is easy to find natural alternatives or make your own with a few simple ingredients. For an all-purpose cleaning spray, try vinegar, castile soap,

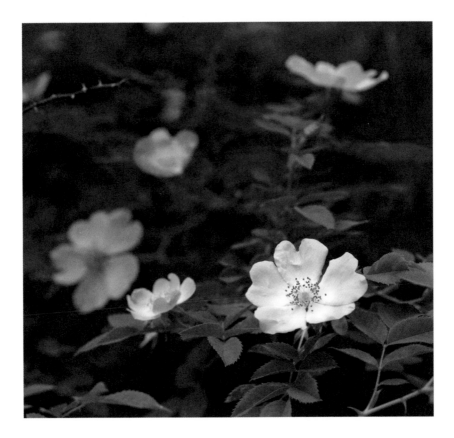

and an essential oil blend. You can also add hydrogen peroxide to make an effective glass cleaner. For scouring, combine baking soda, sea salt, and essential oils.

For laundry, opt for fragrance-free sensitive-skin options from natural brands. To me, nothing is more cloying than the scent of dryer sheets. They cling to your clothes and can cause headaches, respiratory problems, or topical allergic reactions. Plus, the chemicals can enter your bloodstream. For a natural alternative, try adding white or apple cider vinegar to a washcloth and putting it in the dryer. Vinegar prevents static and adds softness to clothes. You can also buy chemical-free reusable dryer sheets or wool dryer balls.

Green Beauty Juice

YIELD: 40 OUNCES

INGREDIENTS

2 cups filtered or distilled water

Juice of 1 lemon

¼ pineapple, peeled and
cut into small pieces

1 cucumber, peeled or unpeeled
as desired, cut into small pieces

1 apple, peeled or unpeeled as
desired, cut into small pieces

4 ribs kale, torn into pieces

ADDITIONAL EQUIPMENT

Powerful blender

Airtight pitcher

This green juice is not only tasty, it is incredibly nutritious for your body both internally and externally. The bromelain in pineapple helps your body synthesize skin-firming collagen. Pineapple is also rich in vitamin C and amino acids that aid with skin-cell repair and rejuvenation. Kale is full of antioxidants, vitamins, and minerals, including vitamin K, which helps heal bruises. Cucumber contains biotin, which is beneficial for strong skin, hair, and nails, and caffeic acid, which helps with swelling, burns, and skin repair. Apples are high in vitamin C, antioxidants, and copper. Lemons not only taste fresh but the juice helps prevent damage caused by free radicals and keeps your face looking fresh, too.

Put all ingredients in blender; process on high speed for 20 seconds.

Store in airtight pitcher in refrigerator for up to 3 days. Drink straight or on ice.

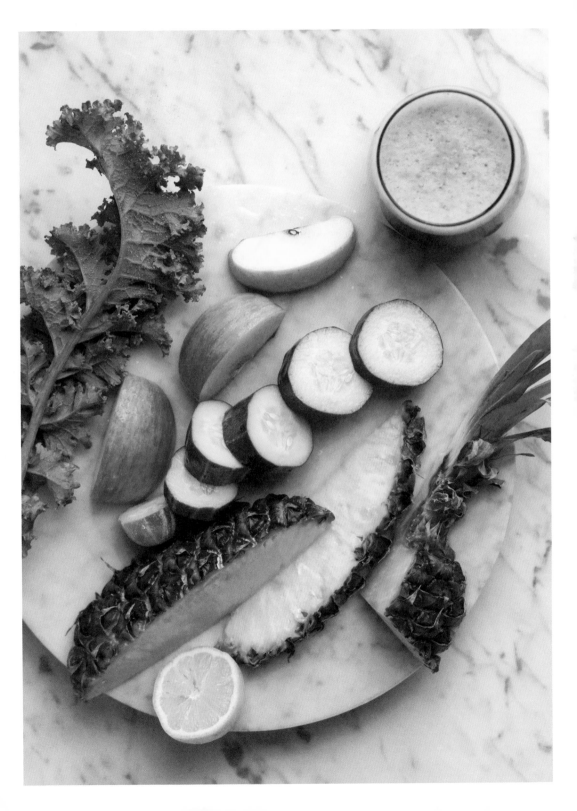

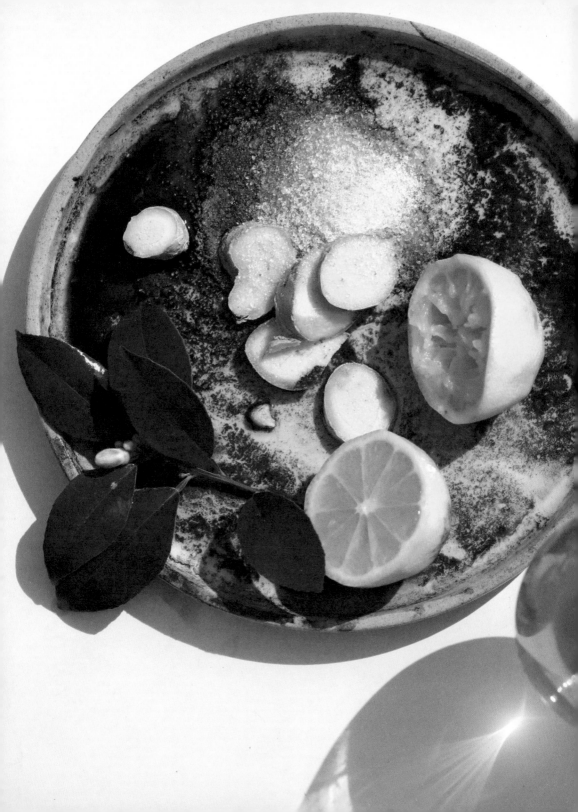

Mer-Made Energy Drink

Spirulina has been harvested and consumed worldwide for its nutritional benefits. It is extremely high in protein, iron, calcium, amino acids, B-complex vitamins, and antioxidants.

With both internal and external benefits, spirulina helps eliminate toxins from the skin, increases skin metabolism to hasten skin-cell turnover, and boosts healing. Known as a natural remedy for acne-prone skin, it helps prevent the growth of candida bacteria that can lead to breakouts.

While this superfood is beautiful in appearance and so rich in goodness for your body, it tastes like pond scum when mixed directly with water. I concocted a recipe that balances the taste and smell of spirulina with fresh lemon, ginger, and sea salt for a refreshing lemonade-like drink I call a Mer-Made. This oceanic-inspired energy-and-health drink is the perfect remedy for dehydration and is full of beneficial nutrients. I like to make a batch and sip it throughout the day. If sour isn't your jam, add a little bit of maple syrup or agave nectar to taste.

YIELD: 32 OUNCES

INGREDIENTS

4 cups filtered or distilled water

Juice of 1 lemon

1 thumb-size knob fresh ginger

¼ teaspoon spirulina

¼ teaspoon sea salt, or Himalayan pink salt

Optional: maple syrup or agave nectar to taste

ADDITIONAL EQUIPMENT

Powerful blender

32-ounce bottle with lid

Put all ingredients in blender; process on low speed for 10 seconds. Best when fresh, but can be stored in refrigerator in lidded bottle for 2 days.

Golden Glow Elixir

YIELD: ABOUT 18 OUNCES

INGREDIENTS

16 ounces raw honey
(local if possible)*

Juice of 3 or 4 lemons

1 large knob fresh ginger*

1 small knob fresh turmeric

* You can also use maple
syrup as a vegan alternative.

** I am a fiery ginger lover,
so feel free to decrease the
ginger as much as you desire.

ADDITIONAL EQUIPMENT

Powerful blender

18-ounce jar with lid

Whenever I get a crick in my throat, I make myself some hot honey-lemon ginger tea. Whenever I get a stomachache, I add the same ingredients to seltzer. This elixir evolved out of that practice. It is an immune-boosting potion packed with alkalizing lemon, anti-inflammatory turmeric, vitality-boosting ginger, and healing local honey. I love it year-round, but especially in the winter, when I need to strengthen my immune system.

To consume:
Take 1 tablespoon daily followed by a glass of water.
Put 1 or 2 tablespoons in hot water to make tea.
Put 1 or 2 tablespoons in seltzer for natural ginger ale.
Use to flavor kombucha.
Use in salad dressing.

———————————————

Pour honey into bowl. Combine lemon juice, ginger, and turmeric in blender; process on medium speed for 30 seconds. Combine with honey. Stir and pour into jar with lid. Liquid will naturally separate; just shake to combine.

Use as desired, but I love to take 1 tablespoon a day. Store in refrigerator for up to 6 months.

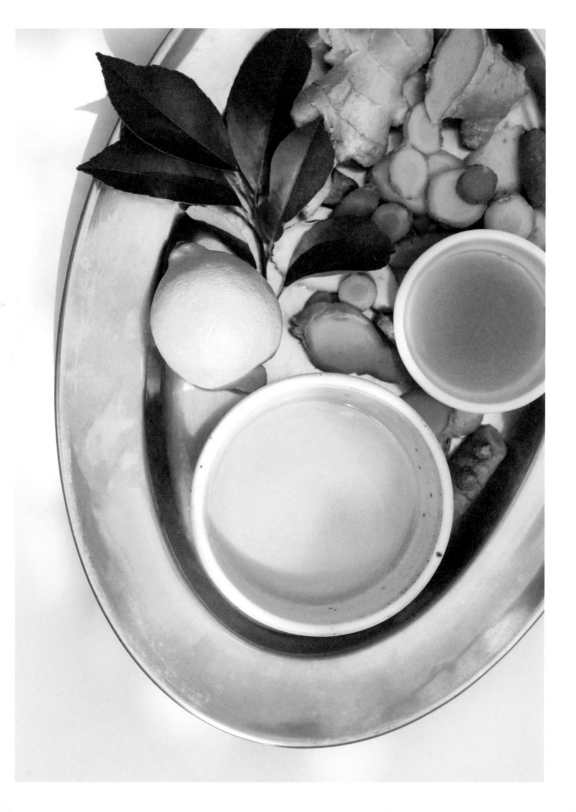

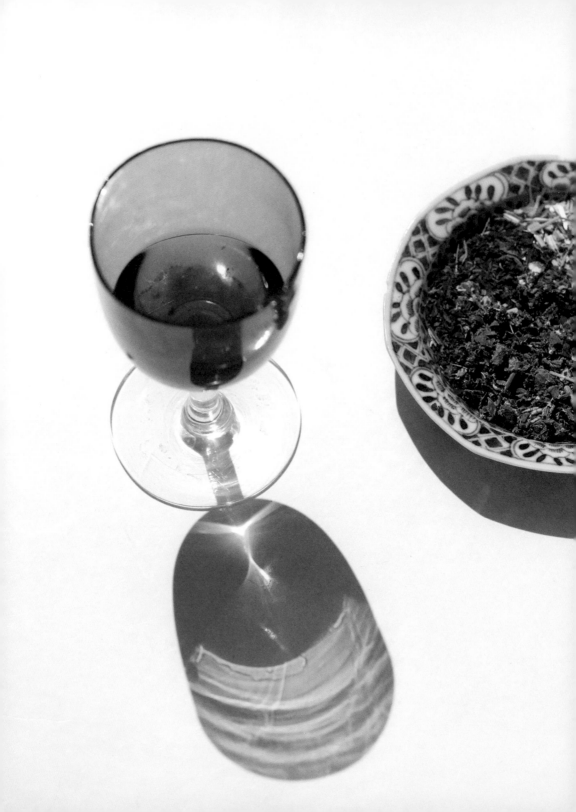

Summer Sun Garden Tea

This is an easy, adaptable recipe that harnesses the power of the sun to make an herbal-infused tea. My favorite herbs to use are mint, lavender, bee balm, lemon balm, lemon verbena, rose petals, and chamomile. This is great on ice.

————————————————

Fill jar with water and add herbs and flowers. Stir well with spoon and put on lid. Leave jar out in a sunny spot for at least 2 hours or up to 6 hours. The longer you infuse, the stronger the tea will be. Strain tea into pitcher and drink immediately.

YIELD: 48 OUNCES

INGREDIENTS

6 cups filtered or distilled water

Approximately 1 cup loosely chopped leaves and flowers from chosen herbs and plants

ADDITIONAL EQUIPMENT

48-ounce Mason jar with lid

Green Sprite Tea

This is a mineralizing and deeply nourishing tea for women's health. Nettle is rich in iron and vitamin K. Raspberry leaf, used to strengthen the uterus, is high in vitamins E and C and helps soothe skin irritation. Oatstraw helps calm the nervous system and aids in healing skin conditions such as eczema and rashes.

————————————————

Combine all ingredients in small bowl and stir. Store in airtight container for up to a year.

To prepare tea, steep 2 teaspoons in 8 ounces boiling water for 10 minutes. Strain and drink. Use daily or as desired.

YIELD: ABOUT 4 OUNCES

INGREDIENTS

2 tablespoons dried lemon balm

1 tablespoon dried nettle leaf

1 tablespoon dried raspberry leaf

2 teaspoons dried oatstraw

2 teaspoons dried chamomile

ADDITIONAL EQUIPMENT

Airtight container

Wild Beauty Tea

YIELD: ¾ CUP

INGREDIENTS

¼ cup dried spearmint leaf

2 tablespoons dried gotu kola

2 tablespoons dried red clover

1 tablespoon dried burdock root

1 tablespoon dried yellow dock

1 tablespoon dried licorice root

ADDITIONAL EQUIPMENT

Airtight container

This tea is not only a powerful blend of gentle detoxifying herbs for body and skin but it actually tastes very good! Each herb was chosen for its distinct properties, and together they form a well-balanced tea that you can drink daily. Yellow dock root probably grows wild in your garden and is a blood purifier, hormone balancer, and a great detoxifying herb, especially for the liver. Burdock root is a blood cleanser that also promotes blood circulation to the skin surface. Red clover detoxifies the liver, blood, and organs as well as balances hormones. In addition to helping promote memory and calm nerves, gotu kola is full of vitamins B and C and has anti-inflammatory properties. Spearmint not only tastes delicious, but it aids digestion, balances hormones, and aids circulation. Licorice root is an adaptogenic herb, helping to maintain the health of the body's adrenal system. In addition to helping balance stress hormones, this herb is also great for gut health.

Combine all ingredients in small bowl and stir. Store in airtight container for up to a year.

To prepare tea, steep 1 tablespoon in 8 ounces boiling water for 8 to 10 minutes. Strain and drink. I recommend drinking at least 1 cup daily.

Petal Tea

This tea was inspired by a petal face mask I created for Captain Blankenship and is a blend of two of my favorite beautiful and beneficial flower petals. Rose and hibiscus are both blooming with powerful anti-inflammatories. Hibiscus is high in vitamin C, helps improve digestion, and helps cool the body. It lends a stunning ruby-red hue to the tea. Sweet rose petals balance the sour taste of hibiscus and add a delicious aroma. This is a favorite everyday tea and one that is delicious and refreshing when chilled.

———————————————

Combine all ingredients in small bowl and stir. Store in airtight container for up to a year.

To prepare tea, steep 1 teaspoon in 8 ounces boiling water for 8 to 10 minutes. Strain and drink. This is also great iced.

YIELD: ABOUT ⅔ CUP

INGREDIENTS

½ cup rose petals

2½ tablespoons hibiscus petals

Optional: 1¼ tablespoons lavender buds

ADDITIONAL EQUIPMENT

Airtight container

Rose & Coconut Water

YIELD: 4 OUNCES

INGREDIENTS

4 ounces raw coconut water

1 teaspoon rose hydrosol

This is a real treat, both hydrating and luscious, that combines the delicate taste of rose paired with the refreshing taste of coconut water. Rose is a remedy for grief and is also a natural aphrodisiac.

―――――――――――――

Combine all ingredients in glass; drink straight or chilled.

Superpower Cocoa Mix

YIELD: 8 OUNCES

INGREDIENTS

½ cup raw cocoa powder

2 tablespoons maca powder

2 tablespoons
ashwagandha powder

2 tablespoons ground
goji berry powder

1 tablespoon ground
schizandra berry powder

ADDITIONAL EQUIPMENT

Airtight container

This isn't your average cocoa; it has super powers. It contains a powerful mix of adaptogenic herbs (maca, ashwagandha, and schizandra) and antioxidant and anti-inflammatory goji berries, as well as raw cocoa powder to help relieve stress, boost energy, and balance hormones. It tastes delicious, too!

For 1 serving, combine 4 ounces boiling water; 1 tablespoon cocoa mix; 2 tablespoons raw milk, nut milk, or coconut milk; and maple syrup or raw honey to taste.

―――――――――――――

Thoroughly mix all ingredients in mixing bowl and spoon into airtight container. Will keep for up to a year.

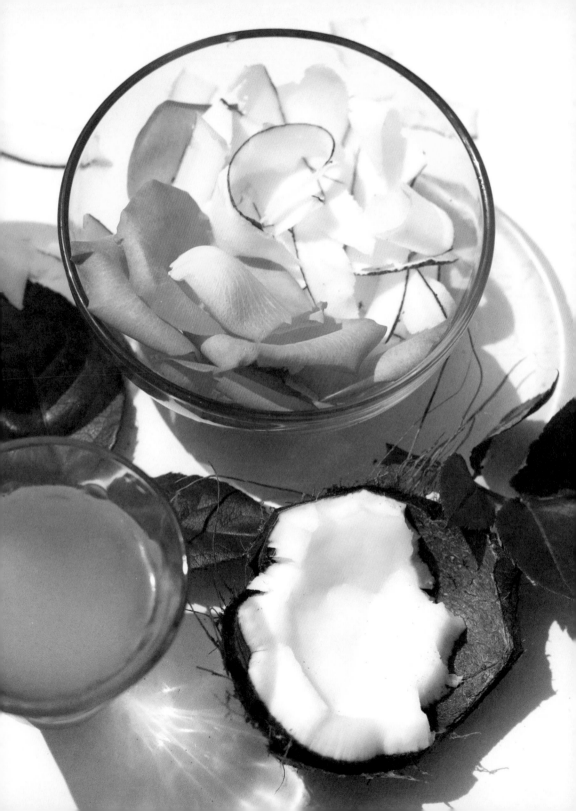

CAPTAIN KIDS

There is an island called Captain Kids right off the coast of
Sorrento. As a child, I found so much wonder encapsulated in this
island. It was the island that was my primary destination on summer days, the one I rowed out to and explored. A wild island with
proud coastal pines encircled by beaches covered in wild thorny
roses and full of seaweed, urchins, and barnacles. As an adult, it is
still special to me and is a symbol of wild nature and wild beauty.
A beautiful children's book called *The Little Island*, by Margaret
Wise Brown, captures the changing of seasons on a tiny island
and the beauty of its being:

> "There was a little Island in the ocean
> Around it the winds blew
> And the birds flew
> And the tides rose and fell on the shore." [18]

In the book, a kitten comes ashore aboard a sailboat and is curi-
ous about what an island is and how it came to be. A fish tells the
kitten that "all land is one land under the sea." [19] As a child, I thought
islands were afloat, but as I grew up, I learned that they are mountains rising up from out of the sea. Somehow knowing this was
comforting, that an island wasn't tossed by the wind but actually
had roots anchored into the ocean. We humans are also not floating
islands but have our own anchors that connect us to the earth.

Afterword

Everything has a beginning, middle, and an end, but the magic lies in the process. I want to return to where I started this book, to childhood. Children live with curiosity, openness, and a profound sense of play. If we can retain our childlike wonder while honoring the elder within, we can move wisely, powerfully, gracefully, intentionally, and playfully in this world. With an eye on the horizon, watching the winds, blue skies, sunrises, sunsets, and the storms brewing, we can stay even keeled and aware. We can be the captain of the ship.

We also need to find our anchor. Let ritual become one of the anchors that colors your days. Think of self-care as you would a meditation practice. Be present and enjoy it. Choose products that make you feel happy and that work for your skin and hair. Make sure to eat well and use herbs as your allies. Know that everything in your being is connected; treat yourself well inside and out. Stay as conscious as possible, and let wild beauty and wild nature guide you in your journey.

It feels powerful to be writing this ending on the summer solstice, the longest day of the year. Outside, bees hum, birds chirp, flowers turn their faces to the sun; everything is green and at its fullest in the summer heat. After the late sunset, the fireflies will create fireworks in our field. Today, I will hike beside mountain laurel blooms to the waterfall and drink my heart's fill of wild nature. On this day, there is so much light flooding the world. In the world, there is so much darkness, injustice, and inhumanity. We need to be the light, to believe in our power and be the radical change.

In nature, we see so many examples of the cycle of life and its beauty. Think about how children revel in the changes in nature that unfold before their eyes: the transformation of a caterpillar to a butterfly, the leaves coming back on bare trees after a long winter, or the bursting open of buds in the summer. Like plants, we humans have deep roots. We are all connected to the earth, for which we are stewards, and to one another. That is why we need to be mindful of what we buy, what we put on our skin and our bodies, and the effect of our scents on those around us and on the environment. Always remember, integrity matters and less is truly more. In the profound words of Mary Oliver, "Attention is the beginning of devotion."[20]

Acknowledgments

Thanks to my superstar team at Ten Speed Press for making this book possible. I am so grateful to my editors, Dervla Kelly and Jenny Wapner, for your openness, support, and feedback. Thanks to my creative director, Emma Campion, and designers, Lisa Ferkel and Isabelle Gioffredi, for bringing this vision to life. Thanks to Jane Chinn in production and Windy Dorresteyn and Lauren Kretzschmar in PR and marketing.

To Mandy Aftel, I am so grateful to you for starting me on this journey, for your friendship and encouragement, and for always being there for me. I am so thankful I stepped into your world of wonder.

To Julianna Blizzard, my photographer and skipper. I am so thankful to have gone on this adventure with you, for your deep respect and love of nature, your creativity and focus in the process, and for the beautiful and wild work you created. You are always an inspiration.

To Chris Lanier, our stylist extraordinaire. Thank you for your hard work and creativity, for getting down and dirty with your ninja skills, always making us laugh and being game for anything. I am so in awe of what you helped us create.

Thanks to Jenny Bowskill and Brad Lail at Lail Design for the beautiful ceramics that we used in the recipe shots.

Thanks to Em Gift for your friendship, support, and for creating the beautiful ceramic shell bowls that we used in the recipe shots.

To my crew at Captain Blankenship (Sara Allexander, Julianna Blizzard, Amy DeAngelis, Karen Holly, Alexandra Dowling Lari, Shannon Mooney, and Magnolia Neel), this ship wouldn't sail without you sisters. Thank you for letting me take the time to step away and work on this book while you kept everything on course. Holy ship, I am lucky to have such an amazing team.

To Lisa Foti-Straus, thank you for being my friend since the beginning of our time in this world, for helping me become who I am, and for supporting me in everything I create in my life.

To Sara Magenheimer, thank you for your deep friendship, your inspiration, and for helping me get this ship sailing from the start. You have always believed in me, supported me, and I am so grateful for our connection.

To Erica Carroll, thank you for being my rainbow for the past twenty-five years and for your support, encouragement, and help always in navigating every part of my life.

To my family (Levi, Mila, Caspian, Ljiljana, Peter, Sasa, Renee, Sofia, Vivienne, Jason, Mira, Andjela, Margaret, Tom, Julika, David, Viola, Xander, Emma, Damon, Laura, and Teddy), I feel your support and love every day.

Thank you to Beth Altshuler, Becca Baker, Rachel Barrett, Erica Beckman, Sara Bright, Amanda Christan Burran, Sarah Cabell, Leandre Camacho, Ajay Chaudhary, Susanrachel Condon, Anna Conlan, Laura Ferrera, Eleanor Friedberger, Chrissy Glenn, Cali Gorewitz, Bronwen Halsey, Patrick Kelly, Katy Kondrat, Maffy Malaver, Eve Mayer, Dana McClure, Cassie McGettigan, Micki Meng, Susannah Morse, Magnolia Neel, Francine Niyonzima, Tara Pelletier, Barrett Purdum, Joanna Radin, Jenn Hoos Rothberg, Romy Silver, Julie Ullman, and Natasha Wheat for your friendship and support. And to all my friends in the green beauty community who have been so welcoming, supportive, and compassionate.

Resources

Many of these products are also available in natural food stores.

HERBS, CARRIER OILS, BUTTERS & WAXES

Jean's Greens
www.jeansgreens.com

Mountain Rose Herbs
www.mountainroseherbs.com

Starwest Botanicals
www.starwest-botanicals.com

ESSENTIAL OILS

Aftelier
www.aftelier.com

Eden Botanicals
www.edenbotanicals.com

Mountain Rose Herbs
www.mountainroseherbs.com

GLASSWARE, EYEDROPPERS & LABWARE

Mountain Rose Herbs
www.mountainroseherbs.com

SKS Bottle & Packaging
www.sks-bottle.com

Specialty Bottle
www.specialtybottle.com

SKIN & BODY CARE

Babo Botanicals
www.babobotanicals.com

Meow Meow Tweet
www.meowmeowtweet.com

Osmia Organics
www.osmiaorganics.com

Earth tu Face
www.earthtuface.com

Odacité
www.odacite.com

S.W. Basics
www.swbasicsofbk.com

Fig & Yarrow
www.figandyarrow.co

Osea Malibu
www.oseamalibu.com

Ursa Major
www.ursamajorvt.com

HAIR CARE

Innersense Beauty
www.innersensebeauty.com

Josh Rosebrook
www.joshrosebrook.com

La Tierra Sagrada
www.latierrasagradahair.com

PERFUME

Aftelier
www.aftelier.com

Ojai Wild
www.ojaiwild.com

Sigil Scent
www.sigilscent.com

Florescent
www.florescent.co

Perfumera Curandera
www.perfumeracurandera.com

Smoke Perfume
www.smokeperfume.com

MAKEUP

Au Naturale
www.aunaturalecosmetics.com

Gressa
www.gressaskin.com

RMS Beauty
www.rmsbeauty.com

Axiology
www.axiologybeauty.com

ILIA Beauty
www.iliabeauty.com

Vapour Organic Beauty
www.vapourbeauty.com

Bibliography

Ackerman, Diane. 1990. *A Natural History of the Senses*. New York: Vintage Books.

Aftel, Mandy. 2001. *Essence and Alchemy*. New York: North Point Press.

——— . 2014. *Fragrant: The Secret Life of Scent*. New York: Riverhead Books.

Artemis, Nadine. 2017. *Renegade Beauty: Reveal and Revive Your Natural Radiance*. Berkeley, CA: North Atlantic Books.

Damian, Peter and Kate. 1995. *Aromatherapy: Scent and Psyche*. Rochester, VT: Healing Arts Press.

Estés, Clarissa Pinkola, 1992. *Women Who Run with the Wolves*. New York: Ballantine Books.

Falconi, Dina. 1998. *Earthly Bodies & Heavenly Hair*. Woodstock, NY: Ceres Press.

——— . *Foraging & Feasting: A Field Guide and Wild Food Cookbook*. Accord, NY: Botanical Arts Press.

Groves, Maria Noel. 2016. *Body into Balance*. North Adams, MA: Storey Publishing.

Herz, Rachel. 2007. *The Scent of Desire*. New York: Harper Collins.

Horowitz, Alexandra. 2009. *Inside of a Dog: What Dogs See, Smell, and Know*. New York: Scribner.

Jansson, Tove. 1954. *Moominsummer Madness*. Translated by Thomas Warburton. New York: Square Fish.

Lawless, Julia. 2013. *The Encyclopedia of Essential Oils*. San Francisco: Conari Press.

Martin, Agnes. 1992. *Writings*. Berlin: Hatje Cantz.

O'Connor, Siobhan, and Alexandra Spunt. 2010. *No More Dirty Looks*. Cambridge, MA: Da Capo Lifelong Books.

Oliver, Mary. 1992. *New and Selected Poems, Volume One*. Boston: Beacon Press.

——— . 2016. *Upstream: Selected Essays*. New York: Penguin Press.

Rose, Jeanne. 1993. *The Aromatherapy Book*. Berkeley, CA: North Atlantic Books.

——— . 1999. *375 Essential Oils and Hydrosols*. Berkeley, CA: North Atlantic Books.

Winter, Ruth. 2009. *A Consumer's Dictionary of Cosmetic Ingredients*. New York: Harmony Books.

Wise Brown, Margaret. 1946. *The Little Island*. New York: Random House.

Notes

1. Martin, Agnes. 1992. *Writings*. Berlin: Hatje Cantz, 35.

2. Aftel, Mandy. 2014. *Fragrant: The Secret Life of Scent*. New York: Riverhead Books, 4.

3. Aftel, 4–5.

4. Ackerman, Diane. 1990. *A Natural History of the Senses*. New York: Vintage Books, 20.

5. Ackerman, 20.

6. Aftel, Mandy. 2001. *Essence and Alchemy*. New York: North Point Press, 37.

7. Damian, Peter and Kate. 1995. *Aromatherapy: Scent and Psyche*. Rochester, VT: Healing Arts Press: 11.

8. Herz, Rachel. 2017. *The Scent of Desire*. New York: HarperCollins, 18–19.

9. Horowitz, Alexandra. 2009. *Inside of a Dog: What Dogs See, Smell, and Know*. New York, Scribner: 71.

10. Jana Blankenship in conversation with Maria Soledad, December 30, 2017.

11. Estés, Clarissa Pinkola. 1992. *Women Who Run with the Wolves*. New York, Ballantine Books: 205.

12. Jansson, Tove. 1954. *Moominsummer Madness*. Translated by Thomas Warburton. New York: Square Fish, 13.

13. Ackerman, 84.

14. Oliver, Mary. 2016. *Upstream: Selected Essays*. New York: Penguin Press, 6.

15. Falconi, Dina. 2013. *Foraging & Feasting: A Field Guide and Wild Food Cookbook*. Accord, NY: Botanical Arts Press, 1.

16. Estés, 11.

17. Estés, 11.

18. Wise Brown, Margaret. 1946. *The Little Island*. New York: Random House, 1.

19. Wise Brown, 29.

20. Oliver, 8.

Index

absolutes, 24
Ackerman, Diane, 20, 117
acne, 92–93
adaptogens, 137
Aftel, Mandy, 17, 19, 37, 133
aloe vera, 67
antioxidants, 91
apple cider vinegar (ACV), 67
    Refreshing Hibiscus ACV Rinse, 123
Aquamarine Bubble Bath, 77
argan, 69
aromatherapy, 29

bacteria, 92
basil, 44
baths
    Aquamarine Bubble Bath, 77
    Emerald Sea Detox Bath, 77
beeswax, 71
beverages
    Golden Glow Elixir, 144
    Green Beauty Juice, 140
    Mer-Made Energy Drink, 143
    Rose & Coconut Water, 150
    Superpower Cocoa Mix, 150
    See also tea
body
    Cocoa-Nut Body Butter, 82
    Hydrating Body Wash, 78
    No-More-Scales Body Oil, 79
    Sea Salt & Sunshine Body Scrub, 84
    Smell the Roses Face Toner &
        Body Mist, 106
Brown, Margaret Wise, 152
butane, 72
Butterfly Daytime Face Oil, 110

caffeine, 135
Calming Blend, Sweet Rest, 54
Calming Spray, Deep Breath, 57
candelilla wax, 71
candles, 31–32
Captain Blankenship
    founding of, 13, 15
    motto of, 15
carbon dioxide extraction, 24
carriers, 28–29, 69–70
castile soap, 68, 74
chamomile, 39, 64
charcoal, activated, 67
citrus oils, 43, 46
clary sage, 41–42
clay, 68
cleaning products, 138–39

cleansing herbs, 137
Clean Slate Makeup Remover &
    Oil-Based Cleanser, 100
Clearing Spray, Good Vibrations, 58
coal tar, 72
cocoa
    Cocoa & Spice Face Mask &
        Exfoliant, 96
    Superpower Cocoa Mix, 150
cocoa butter, 71
    Cocoa-Nut Body Butter, 82
coconut oil, 69–70
collagen, 91
concretes, 24
Cream-Dream Deodorant, 80
Creamy Shea Face Cleanser, 103
creativity, 135
crystals, 136

Deep Breath Calming Spray, 57
Deep Sleep Eye Serum, 109
Deodorant, Cream-Dream, 80
diazolidinyl urea, 72
digestive plants, 138
dry brushing, 64

elastin, 91
Emerald Green Woods Room Spray, 57
Emerald Sea Detox Bath, 77
Energy Drink, Mer-Made, 143
enfleurage, 23–24
equipment, 46
essential oils
    definition of, 19
    extracting, 21–22
    history of, 21
    intensities of, 22
    pregnancy and, 45
    sourcing, 21
    See also individual oils
Estés, Clarissa Pinkola, 61, 133
eucalyptus, 42
Eye Serum, Deep Sleep, 109

face
    Butterfly Daytime Face Oil, 110
    Cocoa & Spice Face Mask &
        Exfoliant, 96
    Creamy Shea Face Cleanser, 103
    Fresh Face Fruit Mask, 99
    Golden Glow Face Balm, 108
    Maine Face Mask, 100
    pH for, 89
    Shimmer & Pop Highlighter, 114
    See also makeup; toners

Falconi, Dina, 130
fir, 42
Fly & Tick Spray, 83
food, 131, 134–35
Forest Sprite Grounding Blend, 54
formaldehyde, 72
frankincense, 31, 37
free radicals, 91
fruit enzymes, 68
Fruit Mask, Fresh Face, 99

Gattefossé, René-Maurice, 29
geranium, 39, 65
Golden Glow Elixir, 144
Golden Glow Face Balm, 108
Good Vibrations Clearing Spray, 58
gratitude, 134
Gravel & Gold, 15
Green Beauty Juice, 140
Green Sprite Tea, 147
Grounding Blend, Forest Sprite, 54

hair
    brushing, 119
    coloring, 119
    exfoliation and, 119
    Mermaid Hair Mask, 120
    Refreshing Hibiscus ACV Rinse, 123
    Sea Salt Wave Spray, 126
    Shining Waves Hair Oil, 125
    styling, 118
    washing, 118
    Witchy Coconut Leave-In
        Conditioner & Detangler, 126
    See also shampoo
Halprin, Anna, 135
herbalism, 130–31, 137–38
Herz, Rachel, 30
Highlighter, Shimmer & Pop, 114
honey, 68
    Milk & Honey Shampoo, 122
Hydrating Body Wash, 78
hydroquinone, 73
hydrosols, 22, 91

immune-boosting plants, 137
incense, 31
ingredients
    to avoid, 72–74
    favorite, 67–71
    organic, 46
    reading lists of, 62–64, 67
    See also individual ingredients
isolates, 24–25

Jansson, Tove, 87
jasmine, 38
    Vine Jasmine Blend, 49
jewelweed, 130
jojoba oil, 70
juniper berry, 42

laundry, 139
lavandin, 39
lavender, 39, 65
lemongrass, 43
lemon verbena, 44
Lips Balm, Lick Your, 113
Loosen the Knot Tension-Release
    Blend, 53

Maine Face Mask, 100
makeup
    Clean Slate Makeup Remover &
        Oil-Based Cleanser, 100
    conventional, 94
maple syrup, 68
memory herbs, 138
Mer-Made Energy Drink, 143
Mermaid Hair Mask, 120
Milk & Honey Shampoo, 122
mint, 43
moisturizers, 93
movement, 135
myrrh, 31, 37

nail polish, 94
natural fragrance, 26, 30
neroli, 39, 41
    Vernal Neroli Blend, 50
No-More-Scales Body Oil, 79

Old Ford Farm, 131
Oliver, Mary, 129, 153
orange blossom, 39, 41

parabens, 73
patchouli, 37
peppermint, 43
perfumes
    creation of, 36
    etymology of, 29
    well-balanced, 36
Perkin, William Henry, 25
Petal Tea, 149
petrochemicals, 73
phthlates, 73
pine, 42
Pollan, Michael, 62

pregnancy, 45
preservatives, 64
probiotics, 92, 135, 137
propylene glycol, 73

Queen Anne's lace, 130

Refreshing Hibiscus ACV Rinse, 123
retinyl palmitate, 73
Room Spray, Emerald Green Woods, 57
rose, 30, 41
    Petal Tea, 149
    Rose & Coconut Water, 150
    Smell the Roses Face Toner &
        Body Mist, 106
    Venus Rose Blend, 50
rose geranium, 39
rosehip seed oil, 70
rosemary, 65
rosewater, 22

Sail-Away Dry Shampoo, 127
sandalwood, 37-38
scent
    extractions, 22-25
    power of, 18-19, 20, 32
sea buckthorn oil, 70
sea salt, 68
    Sea Salt & Sunshine Body Scrub, 84
    Sea Salt Wave Spray, 126
seaweed, 69
sebum, 89
self-care, 132, 153
shampoo
    dry, 119
    Milk & Honey Shampoo, 122
    Sail-Away Dry Shampoo, 127
shea butter, 62, 64, 71
    Creamy Shea Face Cleanser, 103
Shimmer & Pop Highlighter, 114
Shining Waves Hair Oil, 125
skin
    collagen and, 91
    dry, 88, 89, 91
    elastin and, 91
    herbs and, 138
    oil and, 88
    seasonal care for, 93
    sunshine and, 93-94
    See also body; face
sleep, 137
Smell the Roses Face Toner &
    Body Mist, 106
smudging, 31, 32

Soledad, Maria, 35
spearmint, 43
sponges, 64
substitutions, 46
Summer Sun Garden Tea, 147
sunflower seed oil, 70
sunshine, 93-94
Superpower Cocoa Mix, 150
surfactants, 74
Sweet Rest Calming Blend, 54
synthetic fragrance, 25-26, 28, 30, 74

talc, 74
tea
    Fresh Green Tea Clarifying
        Toner, 103
    Green Sprite Tea, 147
    Petal Tea, 149
    Summer Sun Garden Tea, 147
    Wild Beauty Tea, 148
tea tree, 42
Tension-Release Blend, Loosen
    the Knot, 53
toluene, 74
toners, 89, 91
    Fresh Green Tea Clarifying
        Toner, 103
    Smell the Roses Face Toner &
        Body Mist, 106
towels, 64
triclocarban, 74
triclosan, 74

vanilla, 38
Venus Rose Blend, 50
verbena, 44
Vernal Neroli Blend, 50
vetiver, 38
Vine Jasmine Blend, 49

water, 135
Wild Beauty Tea, 148
witch hazel, 69
    Witchy Coconut Leave-In
        Conditioner & Detangler, 126
women's health herbs, 138

ylang ylang, 41
yogurt, 69

Published in the United States by Ten Speed Press,
an imprint of Random House, a division of
Penguin Random House LLC, New York.
www.crownpublishing.com
www.tenspeed.com

Ten Speed Press and the Ten Speed Press colophon are
registered trademarks of Penguin Random House LLC.

Library of Congress Cataloging-in-Publication Data
Names: Blankenship, Jana, author.
Title: Wild beauty : wisdom & recipes for natural self-care / Jana Blankenship.
Description: First edition. | California : Ten Speed Press, [2018] | Includes
    bibliographical references and index. |
Identifiers: LCCN 2018045502 (print) | LCCN 2018047811 (ebook)
Subjects: LCSH: Aromatherapy. | Self-care, Health. | BISAC: HEALTH
    HEALTH & FITNESS/ Beauty & Grooming. | HEALTH & FITNESS / Aromatherapy.
Classification: LCC RM666.A68 (ebook) | LCC RM666.A68 B53 2018 (print)
    615.3/219—dc23
LC record available at https://lccn.loc.gov/2018045502

Hardcover ISBN: 978-0-399-58281-3
eBook ISBN: 978-0-399-58282-0

Printed in China

Design by Isabelle Gioffredi
Prop styling by Chris Lanier

10 9 8 7 6 5 4 3 2 1

First Edition